# Problem Solving in Haematology

# Problem Solving in
# Haematology

**GRAEME SMITH**
Consultant Haematologist, Clinical Director, Department of Haematology,
St James's Institute of Oncology, Leeds, UK

**CLINICAL PUBLISHING**
OXFORD

CLINICAL PUBLISHING

an imprint of Atlas Medical Publishing Ltd
Oxford Centre for Innovation
Mill Street, Oxford OX2 0JX, UK

tel: +44 1865 811116
fax: +44 1865 251550

email: info@clinicalpublishing.co.uk
web: www.clinicalpublishing.co.uk

**Distributed in USA and Canada by:**
Clinical Publishing
30 Amberwood Parkway
Ashland OH 44805 USA
tel: 800-247-6553 (toll free within US and Canada)
fax: 419-281-6883
email: order@bookmasters.com

**Distributed in UK and Rest of World by:**
Marston Book Services Ltd
PO Box 269
Abingdon
Oxon OX14 4YN
UK
tel: +44 1235 465500
fax: +44 1235 465555
email: trade.orders@marston.co.uk

A catalogue record for this book is available from the British Library.

ISBN 13      978 1 84692 005 9
ISBN e-book  978 1 84692 605 1

Project manager: Gavin Smith, GPS Publishing Solutions, Herts, UK
Typeset by Phoenix Photosetting, Chatham, UK
Printed by Marston Book Services, Abingdon, Oxon, UK

# Contents

# Contributors

Prof. David Bowen, Leeds

Dr Gordon Cook, Leeds

Dr Anne Critchley, Leeds

Dr Sylvia Feyler, Huddersfield

Dr Maria Gilleece, Leeds

Dr Di Gilson, Leeds

Dr Quentin Hill, Leeds

Prof. Peter Hillmen, Leeds

Dr Rod Johnson, Leeds

Prof. Sally Kinsey, Leeds

Dr Chris Millar, Middlesborough

Dr Lisa Newton, Bradford

Dr Derek Norfolk, Leeds

Dr Roger Owen, Leeds

Dr Graeme Smith, Leeds

Dr David Swirsky, Leeds

# Abbreviations

| | | | |
|---|---|---|---|
| ABVD | adriamycin, bleomycin, vinblastine and dacarbazine | ChlVPP | chlorambucil, vinblastine, procarbazine and prednisolone |
| ACA | additional chromosome abnormalities | CHOP | cyclophosphamide, adriamycin [doxorubicin], vincristine and prednisolone |
| ACD | anaemia of chronic disease | | |
| ACS | acute chest syndrome | CHR | complete haematologic response |
| ADP | adenosine diphosphate | CIMF | chronic idiopathic myelofibrosis |
| AIHA | autoimmune haemolytic anaemia | CLL | chronic lymphocytic leukaemia |
| ALG | antilymphocyte globulin | CML | chronic myeloid leukaemia |
| ALL | acute lymphoblastic leukaemia | CN | cytogenetically normal |
| alloBMT | allogeneic bone marrow transplantation | CNS | central nervous system |
| | | COPPABVD | cyclophosphamide, vincristine, procarbazine, prednisolone and ABVD |
| alloSCT | allogeneic stem cell transplantation | | |
| ALT | alanine transferase | | |
| AML | acute myeloid leukaemia | CPHPC | R-1-[6-[R-2-carboxy-pyrrolidin-1-yl]-6-oxo-hexanoyl]pyrrolidine-2-carboxylic acid |
| ANA | antinuclear antibody | | |
| ANC | absolute neutrophil count | | |
| APA | antiphospholipid antibodies | CR | complete remission/complete response |
| APC | activated protein C | | |
| APS | antiphospholipid syndrome | CR1 | first complete remission |
| APTT | activated partial thromboplastin time | CRAB | hyperCalcaemia, Renal dysfunction, Anaemia, Bone fractures or lytic lesions |
| ARDS | adult respiratory distress syndrome | | |
| ASCT | autologous stem cell transplantation | CSA | ciclosporin |
| | | CSF | cerebrospinal fluid |
| ATG | antithymocyte globulin | CSSCD | Cooperative Study of Sickle Cell Disease |
| AVN | avascular necrosis | | |
| BCSH | British Committee for Standards in Haematology | CT | computed tomography |
| | | CVP | central venous pressure |
| BEACOPP | bleomycin, etoposide, adriamycin [doxorubicin], cyclophosphamide, vincristine, procarbazine and prednisolone | CVP | cyclophosphamide, vincristine and prednisolone |
| | | CXR | chest X-ray |
| | | CyR | cytogenetic response |
| BEAM | carmustine, etoposide, cytarabine and melphalan | DCT | direct Coombs' test |
| | | DDAVP | 1-deamino-8-D-arginine vasopressin |
| BMT | bone marrow transplantation | | |
| CALGB | Cancer and Leukemia Group B | DEXA | dual-energy X-ray absorptiometry |
| CAP | cyclophosphamide, adriamycin [doxorubicin] and prednisolone | DFS | disease-free survival |
| | | DIC | disseminated intravascular coagulation |
| CCyR | complete cytogenetic response | | |
| 2-CDA | 2-chlorodeoxyadenosine (cladribine) | DLBCL | diffuse large B-cell non-Hodgkin lymphoma |
| CEL | chronic eosinophilic leukaemia | DVT | deep vein thrombosis |

| | | | |
|---|---|---|---|
| EBMT | European Blood and Marrow Transplantation | HPA | human platelet antigen |
| | | HR | haematologic response |
| EDTA | ethylenediaminetetraacetic acid | HU | hydroxyurea |
| EFS | event-free survival | HUS | haemolytic uremic syndrome |
| EMEA | European Medicines Agency | ICH | intracranial haemorrhage |
| EP | extramedullary plasmacytomas | IFRT | involved field radiotherapy |
| EPO | erythropoietin | Ig | immunoglobulin |
| ESP | erythropoiesis-stimulating protein | IL | interleukin |
| ESR | erythrocyte sedimentation rate | IMF | idiopathic myelofibrosis |
| ET | essential thrombocythaemia | IMiD | immunomodulatory drug |
| FAB | French–American–British | INR | International Normalized Ratio |
| FBC | full blood count | IPI | International Prognostic Index |
| FC | fludarabine combined with cyclophosphamide | IPSS | International Prognostic Scoring System |
| FDG-PET | $^{18}$F-fluoro-deoxyglucose positron emission tomography | IR | imatinib-responsive |
| | | ITD | internal tandem duplication |
| FFP | fresh frozen plasma | ITP | idiopathic thrombocytopenic purpura |
| FI | full intensity | | |
| FISH | fluorescent *in situ* hybridization | ITU | intensive therapy unit |
| FIX | factor IX | IV | intravenous |
| FL | follicular lymphoma | JVP | jugular venous pressure |
| FLC | free light chain | LDH | lactate dehydrogenase |
| FLIPI | Follicular Lymphoma International Prognostic Index | LMWH | low-molecular-weight heparin |
| | | LPD | lymphoproliferative disease |
| FNA | fine needle aspirate | LVF | left ventricular failure |
| FV | factor V | M4Eo | acute myeloid leukaemia with eosinophilia |
| FVIII | factor VIII | | |
| FX | factor X | MCH | mean corpuscular haemoglobin |
| FXI | factor XI | MCHC | mean corpuscular haemoglobin concentration |
| G-CSF | granulocyte colony-stimulating factor | | |
| | | MCV | mean cell volume |
| GFR | glomerular filtration rate | MDS | myelodysplastic syndrome |
| GI | gastrointestinal | β2-MG | β2-microglobulin |
| GIFAbs | growth inhibitory factor antibodies | MGUS | monoclonal gammopathy of undetermined significance |
| GP | General Practitioner | | |
| GPI | glycosyl phosphatidyl inositol | MmolR | major molecular response |
| GvHD | graft-versus-host disease | MP | melphalan and prednisone |
| GvL | graft-versus-leukaemia | MPL | thrombopoietin receptor |
| GvM | graft-versus-myeloma | MR | minimal response |
| Hb | haemoglobin | MRC | Medical Research Council |
| HbF | haemoglobin F | MRD | minimal residual disease |
| HbS | haemoglobin S | MRI | magnetic resonance imaging |
| HCT | haematocrit | MSH | Multicenter Study of Hydroxyurea in Sickle Cell Anemia |
| HDAC | histone deacetylase | | |
| HDMTX | high-dose methotrexate | MT | massive transfusion |
| HES | hypereosinophilic syndrome | MUD | matched unrelated donor |
| HIT | heparin-induced thrombocytopenia | nCR | near-complete response |
| HIV | human immunodeficiency virus | NHL | non-Hodgkin lymphoma |
| HLA | human leukocyte antigen | NPM | nucleophosmin |
| HNA | human neutrophil antigen | OS | overall survival |

| | | | |
|---|---|---|---|
| PBSC | peripheral blood stem cell | sIg | surface immunoglobulin |
| PBSCT | peripheral blood stem cell transplantation | SLE | systemic lupus erythematosis |
| | | SM | systemic mastocytosis |
| PCI | protein creatinine index | SVCO | superior vena cava obstruction |
| PCM | plasma cell myeloma | TACO | transfusion associated circulatory overload |
| PCNSL | primary central nervous system lymphoma | TBI | total body irradiation |
| PCR | polymerase chain reaction | TEDS | thromboembolic deterrent stockings |
| PCyR | partial cytogenetic response | | |
| PEG | polyethylene glycol | TF | tissue factor |
| PET | positron emission tomography | TIPSS | transjugular intrahepatic portosystemic shunt |
| PFA | platelet function analyser | | |
| PMF | primary myelofibrosis | TKI | tyrosine kinase inhibitor |
| PNH | paroxysmal nocturnal haemoglobinuria | TOPPS | Trial of Platelet Prophylaxis |
| | | TRALI | transfusion-related acute lung injury |
| PR | partial remission/partial response | | |
| PSA | polysialic acids | TRM | transplant-related mortality |
| PT | prothrombin time | TT | thrombin time |
| PTD | partial tandem duplication | TTP | thrombotic thrombocytopenic purpura |
| PV | polycythaemia vera | | |
| RA | refractory anaemia | UCB | umbilical cord blood |
| RARS | refractory anaemia with ringed sideroblasts | UFH | unfractionated heparin |
| | | VAD | vincristine, adriamycin (doxorubicin) and dexamethasone |
| RBC | red blood cell | | |
| RCT | randomized controlled trial | | |
| rFVIIa | recombinant factor VIIa | VBMCP | vincristine, carmustine, melphalan, cyclophosphamide and prednisone |
| rhEPO | recombinant human erythropoietin | | |
| RIC | reduced-intensity conditioning | vCJD | variant Creutzfeldt Jacob Disease |
| ROTI | myeloma-related organ and/or tissue impairment | VKOR | vitamin K epoxide reductase |
| | | VTE | venous thromboembolism |
| RT–PCR | reverse transcription–polymerase chain reaction | VWF | von Willebrand factor |
| | | WBC | white blood cell |
| SAP | serum amyloid P | WBRT | whole brain radiotherapy |
| SBP | solitary bone plasmacytomas | WCC | white cell count |
| SC | subcutaneous | WHO | World Health Organization |
| SCD | sickle cell disease | WM | Waldenström's macroglobulinaemia |
| SCT | stem cell transplantation | ZPI | protein Z-dependent protease inhibitor |
| SHOT | Serious Hazards of Transfusion | | |

# Introduction

**PROBLEM**

## 01 The approach to the patient with an abnormal blood count

## Case History

 A 47-year-old female consults her doctor complaining of a sore throat of two weeks' duration, and has been aware of bruising affecting her forearms, thighs and shins, apparently developing spontaneously, for a week. She consults her General Practitioner who performs a full blood count.

**What information may be gleaned from this investigation that may aid diagnosis in this case?**

## Background

 The full blood count (FBC) is one of the most common investigations requested by doctors, and an abnormal FBC may be the first indication that a patient may have one of the primary haematological disorders discussed in this book. The test is the cornerstone of haematological diagnosis and the main test performed in haematology laboratories. Between 500 and 700 such tests will be performed daily in an average-sized district general hospital in the UK. The FBC is generated by automated instruments that count and size circulating blood cells by a variety of methods, one of the most common being 'aperture impedance' – the number and volume of cells are proportional to the frequency and height of electric pulses generated when cells pass through a small aperture. It is by this method, for example, that the mean cell volume (MCV) of red cells is determined. These machines also measure directly the haemoglobin content of the red cells, by spectrophotometric analysis after the red cells are lysed, and the haematocrit. As well as these directly measured parameters there are other calculated variables including the mean corpuscular haemoglobin (MCH) and the mean corpuscular haemoglobin concentration

(MCHC). Furthermore, such analysers can provide additional information about the various categories of white blood cells (WBCs) through complex multiparameter analysis of cell size and content, for example by assessing myeloperoxidase content that is found in neutrophils.

In interpreting a FBC, the most significant parameters to focus on are the haemoglobin – which may indicate the presence of anaemia or polycythaemia; the MCV – which will help in the classification of anaemias (see Chapter 7); the white cell count with differential – which would be important in the diagnosis of lymphoid or myeloid disorders; and a platelet count. The interpretation of any abnormality should be made in light of the knowledge that 5% of the population will display laboratory values outside the so-called normal range, and that well-recognized differences in these variables can be observed in persons of different race and between the sexes. For example, persons of African descent may have a lower white cell count (WCC), especially neutrophils, than Caucasians.[1]

### Red cells – anaemia and polycythaemia

The approach to the anaemic patient is described further in Section 3, and polycythaemia in Section 6, and will not be further discussed here. The rest of this chapter will focus instead on the interpretation of an abnormal white cell or platelet count.

The history of a sore throat in this case suggests the possibility of recent infection, and the WCC may be expected to be abnormal, either as a reactive phenomenon or where there may possibly be a causative association.

### White cells – leucopenia

In patients with an abnormal WCC, a 'five population' differential count should immediately tell the clinician which cell line – be it neutrophils, lymphocytes, monocytes, eosinophils or basophils – is affected.

### Neutropenia

Neutropenia becomes clinically relevant only when it is severe (absolute neutrophil count [ANC] $<0.5 \times 10^9$/l) at which point there is a measurable increase in the risk of infection[2] (neutropenia of this degree is conventionally classified into congenital and acquired categories though, as already stated, 'ethnic' neutropenia in people of African origin needs to be recognized early on in the assessment of a patient). Congenital neutropenia includes Kostmann's syndrome and cyclical neutropenia.

The most frequent cause of acquired neutropenia is drug therapy (Table 1.1) with a long list of potential offenders. In the clinical assessment of the patient the possibility of a drug-induced neutropenia means that any possible contributing drug should, if at all possible, be stopped immediately. In this setting, early use of granulocyte colony-stimulating factor (G-CSF) should be considered. Autoimmune conditions and various haematological malignancies enter the differential diagnosis. Many of these conditions are suggested by the clinical assessment of the patient but further investigations, including peripheral blood immunophenotyping, and bone marrow examination may be required.[3]

### Lymphopenia

Lymphopenia is most commonly seen in the setting of recent therapy with immunosuppressive drugs including corticosteroids. Recent viral infection is also a common cause

| Table 1.1 Drugs associated with neutropenia[4] | |
|---|---|
| Anticonvulsants | e.g. phenytoin |
| Antithyroid agents | e.g. carbimazole |
| Phenothiazines | e.g. carbamazepine |
| Anti-inflammatories | e.g. phenylbutazone |
| Antibacterials | e.g. co-trimoxazole |
| Others | e.g. gold, penicillamine, tolbutamide, mianserin, imipramine, cytotoxics |

and consideration should be given to autoimmune and connective tissue disease, sarcoidosis and chronic renal failure.

## White cells – leucocytosis

In any patient in whom an elevated WCC is detected it is essential to examine the blood film, which would be part of standard practice in most laboratories. This simple step should immediately identify rare causes such as chronic myeloid leukaemia (CML), chronic lymphocytic leukaemia (CLL) or the various subtypes of acute leukaemia based on the proportion of immature precursors (including blasts), or cells of lymphoid lineage.

## Neutrophilia

This is either a reactive phenomenon or is due to a myeloid malignancy. It is probably the commonest abnormality seen in the white cell series and the list of possible contributions is as long as the list of inflammatory and infective disorders that can affect the human body. Rarer causes such as CML are suggested by an increase in basophils, and also a so-called 'myelocyte peak' where the myelocytes represent the second-most numerous cell after the neutrophil in the white cell differential. In such cases it is very simple to perform fluorescent *in situ* hybridization (FISH) analysis or a polymerase chain reaction (PCR) test to look for the *BCR-ABL* fusion gene associated with this condition.

## Eosinophilia

As in all cases of increased white cell production, secondary or reactive causes are the most common; in this case, parasitic infection, drugs and conditions such as asthma and other allergic conditions (see Chapter 5).

## Monocytosis

A persistent monocytosis, although commonly encountered in viral and fungal infections, may be associated with myeloproliferative disorders and if, in addition, there are morphological abnormalities of white cell maturation such as hypogranular neutrophils and so-called pseudo-Pelger cells, the possibility of chronic myelomonocytic leukaemia (one of the myelodysplastic syndromes) should be considered.

## Lymphocytosis

In evaluating a lymphocytosis, a blood film again would be helpful in distinguishing reactive lymphocytoses such as that associated with glandular fever (and characterized by the

presence of atypical lymphocytes) from, for example, large granular lymphocyte proliferations which may be either reactive or part of a T-cell disorder. A very high lymphocyte
count, with the presence of smear cells, is highly suggestive of CLL though peripheral blood
immunophenotyping is required to define the specific lymphoproliferative disorder.

## Basophilia

This is extremely rare. Reactive increases are sometimes seen in infections and lymphoproliferative disorders and an elevated count is of diagnostic and prognostic importance
in CML.

For the woman described in the case history, the FBC result was as follows:
- Haemoglobin: 12.8 g/dl
- WCC: $6.5 \times 10^9$/l (neutrophils $3.5 \times 10^9$/l, lymphocytes $2.0 \times 10^9$/l, monocytes $0.6 \times 10^9$/l, eosinophils $0.4 \times 10^9$/l)
- Platelets: $10 \times 10^9$/l

**What is the interpretation of this result?**

The patient has a normal haemoglobin level and WCC. The only abnormality is an isolated low platelet count (thrombocytopenia).

## Platelets – thrombocytopenia

The most important first step is to exclude a spuriously low platelet count which may be
induced by ethylenediaminetetraacetic acid (EDTA) clumping of platelets. This is clarified
by examination of the blood film and, if there is any doubt, repeating the FBC using citrate
as an anticoagulant. However, this explanation of a low platelet count would not be associated with any evidence of clinical bleeding, as appears to be the case here. Generally
speaking, the cause of a low platelet count will be either increased consumption or
reduced production. It is also important to consider physiological states such as pregnancy that can be associated with moderate thrombocytopenia (levels as low as $75 \times 10^9$/l),
but the platelet count in this case is much lower than would be expected if this was the
cause. Increased consumption may be due to disordered autoimmunity in the case of
immune thrombocytopenia, which may be idiopathic or related to drugs or infections.
Other disorders that can increase platelet consumption include thrombotic thrombocytopenic purpura (TTP) – examination of the blood film to look for red cell fragmentation
will help exclude this diagnosis – and platelet consumption as part of a wider derangement
of coagulation such as occurs in disseminated intravascular coagulation (DIC). The clinical assessment of the patient will help exclude causes such as hypersplenism or cirrhosis
and, as in the case of neutropenia, drug causes should be considered, some of the commonest culprits being medications given for cardiac disorders, including quinidine and
thiazide diuretics. In a hospital setting, heparin-induced thrombocytopenia (HIT) is an
important cause with significant consequences which needs early consideration and
exclusion. The commonest cause of a low platelet count, that is immune (idiopathic)
thrombocytopenic purpura (ITP), is often a diagnosis of exclusion but, if thought to be
the explanation, contributing underlying disorders such as autoimmune disease, lymphoproliferative disorders and human immunodeficiency virus (HIV) infection need to be

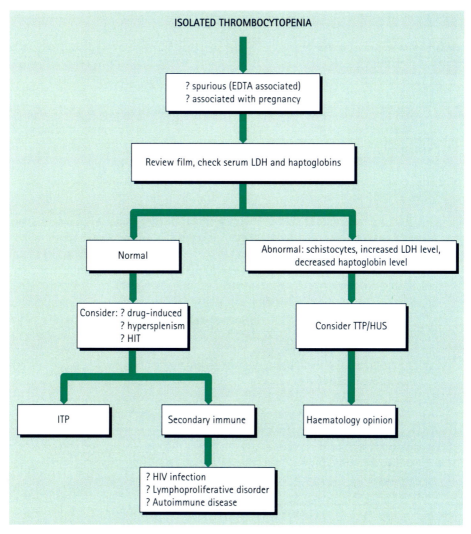

ISOLATED THROMBOCYTOPENIA

? spurious (EDTA associated)
? associated with pregnancy

Review film, check serum LDH and haptoglobins

Normal

Abnormal: schistocytes, increased LDH level, decreased haptoglobin level

Consider: ? drug-induced
? hypersplenism
? HIT

Consider TTP/HUS

ITP

Secondary immune

Haematology opinion

? HIV infection
? Lymphoproliferative disorder
? Autoimmune disease

**Figure 1.1** The approach to a patient with an isolated low platelet count.[5] HUS, haemolytic uremic syndrome; LDH, lactate dehydrogenase.

considered. The condition may develop following viral infections and the history of sore throat in this case may be relevant. Rarer causes of isolated thrombocytopenia include congenital abnormalities such as the May–Hegglin anomaly and Bernard–Soulier syndrome. Both are associated with large (giant) platelets on the blood film. Figure 1.1 summarizes the clinical approach to making a diagnosis, described by Tefferi *et al.*[5]

## Platelets – thrombocytosis

This is usually a secondary process, again related to inflammatory conditions but also to blood loss, asplenia and infection, and hence highlights the importance of taking a full history. The differential diagnosis is primary thrombocythaemia, which may be associated with the Janus kinase 2 (*JAK2*) mutation (see Section 6).

## Recent Developments

The increased sophistication of automated blood counters and parallel advances in auto-mated biochemistry analysers have led many hospitals to house such high throughput instrumentation in joint 'core' laboratories often with the employment of a 'track-based' system in which samples move through the laboratory from a common specimen recep-tion, where once they were sent to separate areas for analysis. Allied to this is the cross-training of staff to form a fully integrated blood sciences diagnostic facility, with increased capacity and allowing the redeployment of staff to more specialist laboratory areas.

## Conclusion

The FBC is a routine part of the assessment of most patients presenting with clinical symptoms to their doctor. It is a lead-in to the majority of the blood disorders described in this book and sensible interpretation of the abnormalities in a logical way can expedite the appropriate referral and management of these cases. The key message is that the FBC findings are always reviewed in the context of the clinical history and examination. This should lead to prompt haematology consultation for those patients who need it, but equally should lead the general physician to perhaps consider non-haematological condi-tions and appropriate referral elsewhere based on a logical interpretation of the abnor-malities that the FBC has uncovered.

In this case the test indicated immediately that the patient's bruising was due to a low platelet count. The normal haemoglobin, MCV, WCC and differential pointed to a diag-nosis of ITP, and this was subsequently confirmed by bone marrow examination. There was no clinical or other evidence of an underlying lymphoproliferative disorder or autoimmune disease and it was likely that this ITP was precipitated by viral infection. Given the significant bruising, treatment was instigated with oral prednisolone 1 mg/kg, with recovery of platelets to normal within 3 days. No recurrence of thrombocytopenia occurred on tailing off steroids after 6 weeks.

## Further Reading

1 Bain BJ. Ethnic and sex differences in the total and differential white cell count and platelet count. *J Clin Pathol* 1996; **49**: 664–6.

2 Bodey GP, Buckley M, Sathe YS, Freireich EJ. Quantitative relationships between circulating leukocytes and infection in patients with acute leukemia. *Ann Intern Med* 1966; **64**: 328–40.

3 van Staa TP, Boulton F, Cooper C, Hagenbeek A, Inskip H, Leufkens HG. Neutropenia and agranulocytosis in England and Wales: incidence and risk factors. *Am J Hematol* 2003; **72**: 248–54.

4 Provan D, Singer CRJ, Baglin T, Lilleyman J. *Oxford Handbook of Clinical Haematology*, 2nd edition. Oxford: Oxford University Press, 2004.

5 Tefferi A, Hanson AC, Inwards DJ. How to interpret and pursue an abnormal complete blood count in adults. *Mayo Clinic Proc* 2005; **80**: 923–36.

# Haemostasis and Thrombosis

**PROBLEM**

# 02  Anticoagulation

## Case History

A 39-year-old woman develops an extensive femoral vein thrombosis. She is receiving chemotherapy for carcinoma of the breast complicated by liver metastases. Haemoglobin is 11.1 g/dl, white cell count $9.2 \times 10^9$/l and platelet count $333 \times 10^9$/l. Her coagulation screen is normal, but liver function tests are abnormal with an obstructive picture.

**How would you manage this case?**

## Background

Optimal management of anticoagulation can be a complex area. Ideally patients should have their treatment individually tailored taking into account the risks and benefits of particular therapies and complicating factors such as comorbid conditions and thrombophilia. These issues are well illustrated by the management of venous thromboembolism (VTE) in patients with cancer.

Venous thromboembolism is a common complication for cancer patients, with a reported incidence of approximately 15%. However, this figure is likely to be much higher as VTE may produce few if any symptoms, which are often attributed to the underlying malignancy. Venous thromboembolism represents an important cause of morbidity and mortality. Data have been published which estimate that one in every seven patients with cancer who require hospital admission and die, do so from a pulmonary embolus.[1]

The risk of VTE in cancer patients is highest in the first few months after diagnosis and is compounded by associated surgery, immobilization, hormone therapy, chemotherapy and central venous catheter insertion. The complications of cancer and its treatment make the management of VTE in such patients a challenge.

## Initial therapy

The use of fixed-dose low-molecular-weight heparin (LMWH) has become standard practice in the initial treatment of VTE. This represents a significant therapeutic advance in terms of ease and convenience of administration. Its longer half-life and increased subcutaneous bioavailability compared with unfractionated heparin (UFH) mean that it can be administered as a single daily dose, lending itself to outpatient treatment and home therapy. There is a lower incidence of heparin-induced thrombocytopenia (HIT) compared with UFH and minimal monitoring is required.

There is still a place for UFH in initial treatment of VTE. In the cancer patient, intravenous UFH may be more appropriate if rapid reversal is required for procedures or in the face of renal impairment. Heparin is cleared by the reticuloendothelial system and renal route. Both mechanisms are important for UFH, but renal clearance predominates for LMWH. This is clinically important as accumulation of LMWH may occur in renal failure, causing an increased bleeding risk.

Long-term heparin use can cause osteoporosis but the absolute risk of symptomatic osteoporosis is unknown. Symptomatic vertebral fractures have been reported in approximately 2%–3% of patients receiving treatment doses of UFH for more than 1 month. The mechanism by which heparin exerts its effects on bone appears to be a decrease in osteoblast activity as well as an increase in osteoclast activity. An animal model has shown that the effects of heparin on bone are reversible but that this is a slow process because heparin binds to bone matrix proteins. Evidence now suggests that LMWHs are associated with a lower risk of osteoporosis than UFH.[2]

The following may be helpful to clinicians when deciding on which heparin preparation and what dose to use:[3]

- the patient's haemostatic potential and hence the intrinsic patient risk of thrombosis or bleeding (patient risk);
- the risk of thrombosis and bleeding associated with the procedure or condition of the patient (disorder risk);
- the relative efficacy of different heparin preparations and doses and the relative bleeding risk associated with these (heparin risk).

Monitoring is not routinely recommended for thromboprophylaxis or treatment with a LMWH but should be considered in certain subgroups, which include the very obese, those with severe renal failure and those in whom the pharmacokinetics of LMWHs may differ, such as infants younger than 3 months and in pregnancy. The activated partial thromboplastin time (APTT) is generally insensitive to LMWHs and cannot be used to monitor dose if this is required. The anti-Xa assay can be helpful but has significant limitations. The following issues need to be considered: the degree of anticoagulation induced by different LMWHs may not be comparable at the same plasma anti-Xa concentration; the comparability between commercially available assays is poor; and the anti-Xa assay appears to have poor correlation with bleeding or thrombosis in subjects receiving a LMWH. Accepting the limitations, monitoring 4–6 hour peak levels using the anti-Xa assay may provide some guidance on dosage. In situations where LMWH may accumulate, such as in renal failure, a trough level may be useful.

The Control of Anticoagulation Subcommittee for the International Society for Thrombosis and Haemostasis has made the following recommendations on monitoring of heparin:[4]

1  Monitoring of prophylactic doses of UFH is not required.
2  Monitoring of prophylactic doses of LMWH is not required routinely. Anti-Xa assay can be employed to detect drug accumulation and risk of overdose in severe renal failure.
3  Monitoring of therapeutic doses of LMWH is not required routinely.
4  Monitoring of therapeutic doses of UFH can be achieved using the APTT. However, local calibration of the test should be employed to determine the recommended target APTT ratio.
5  Use of anti-Xa assays may provide some clue to the pharmacokinetics of LMWH when used to treat thrombosis in those in whom standard or weight-adjusted dosing is likely to be unreliable, especially subjects with severe renal failure, the obese, the pregnant, neonates and infants. Anti-Xa assay may also be of some value in the investigation of unexpected bleeding in a subject receiving a LMWH.
6  Where anti-Xa assay is employed to monitor LMWH therapy, local laboratory assay validation for the heparin in use is important and the limited predictive value of the results in terms of antithrombotic efficiency and bleeding risk of LMWH should be appreciated.

Recommendations 1–3 are based on results of randomized clinical trials of heparin/LMWH prophylaxis or treatment and are grade A. Recommendations 4–6 are based on observational and scientific data.

## Long-term therapy

There are several factors to be considered in the long term. These include future antineoplastic treatment (chemotherapy, hormone therapy), presence of indwelling venous catheters, haemorrhagic risk, increased likelihood of resistance to warfarin, hepatic or renal dysfunction and the prognosis/risk of cancer recurrence.

On anticoagulant treatment, cancer patients have a two- to fourfold higher risk of VTE recurrence and major bleeding compared with cancer-free patients.[5] The increased VTE recurrence is likely to be secondary to the release of cancer procoagulants which are not inhibited by conventional anticoagulation.

Use of LMWH is convenient, flexible and does not pose a problem if there are nutrition difficulties or liver impairment but the risk of osteoporosis is not insignificant. Antivitamin K drugs such as coumarins can prove difficult to control, with an increased risk of over-anticoagulation and haemorrhage. However, the rate of VTE and bleeding is only increased in those patients with advanced disease when compared to non-cancer patients so warfarin could be an option for those with less advanced cancer.[5] Optimal treatment duration is for as long as the malignant disorder is active; this is lifelong for many patients.

There is some evidence for lowered cancer mortality in patients on heparin therapy and this raises the possibility of an antineoplastic effect and the possibility of cancer and thrombosis sharing a common mechanism. The increase in survival has been most strongly linked to lung cancer. Animal models have demonstrated that UFH and LMWH interfere with processes related to tumour growth and metastasis. Retrospective meta-analysis of heparin trials shows that LMWH has been particularly associated with a trend in reducing mortality. This observation has now also been made in some small, prospective studies in which patients without VTE were randomized to a LMWH or placebo, in addition to chemo-radiotherapy.[6,7] The mechanism of action remains unclear and long-term benefit has not yet been proven. Future studies are required to confirm a beneficial effect and address issues such as patient selection, dose and duration of therapy.

In patients with cancer and acute VTE, dalteparin was more effective than an oral anti-coagulant in reducing the risk of recurrent thromboembolism without increasing the risk of bleeding.[8]

The British Committee for Standards in Haematology[3,9] recommends LMWH as first-line treatment for VTE in cancer patients but, in addition, states that heparins are not recommended for use as antineoplastic agents outside clinical trials.

Nine days after starting therapeutic-dose LMWH, the patient develops clinical signs of pulmonary emboli and extension of the deep vein thrombosis (DVT). This is confirmed radiologically. Haemoglobin is 11.3 g/dl, white cell count $12.2 \times 10^9$/l and platelet count $56 \times 10^9$/l.

**What important issues need to be addressed?**

The marked drop in platelet count makes HIT a strong possibility. The management of the patient needs to reflect both this and how to manage the progression of her thrombosis.

## Heparin-induced thrombocytopenia

Heparin-induced thrombocytopenia is a severe complication of heparin treatment occurring with a frequency of 2.6% with UFH and 0.2% with LMWH.[10] The cause of HIT is an antibody which is directed towards the complex formed between heparin and platelet factor 4; this activates platelets and endothelial cells thereby inducing a pro-thrombotic state.

Heparin-induced thrombocytopenia can be associated with UFH, LMWH at prophylactic and therapeutic doses and even by the small amounts of heparin used to flush lines or impregnated in central venous catheters.

The platelet count classically falls 5–10 days after starting heparin, although in patients who have received heparin in the previous 3 months it may occur sooner because of pre-existing antibodies. The onset is rare after more than 15 days of exposure. The platelet count typically falls by >50% with a median nadir of $55 \times 10^9$/l and a platelet count of $<15 \times 10^9$/l is unusual. On average, half of the patients who develop HIT will have associated thrombosis. Those patients presenting without thrombosis have a high risk of subsequent thrombosis if heparin is not discontinued.

The probability of HIT should initially be judged on clinical grounds. There are four factors that are particularly helpful in assessing the likelihood of HIT. These are the degree of thrombocytopenia, the timing of the onset, the presence of new or progressive thrombosis and whether an alternative cause of thrombocytopenia is likely. A scoring system has been devised to assess the pre-test probability (Table 2.1).[11,12] If the pre-test

**Table 2.1** Pre-test probability scoring system for heparin-induced thrombocytopenia

| | Points (0, 1 or 2 for each of four categories: maximum possible score = 8) | | |
| --- | --- | --- | --- |
| | 2 | 1 | 0 |
| Thrombocytopenia | >50% fall or platelet nadir 20–100 × 10⁹/l | 30%–50% fall or platelet nadir 10–19 × 10⁹/l | <30% fall or platelet nadir <10 × 10⁹/l |
| Timing* of platelet count fall or other sequelae | Clear onset between days 5 and 10; or less than 5 days (if heparin exposure within past 100 days) | Consistent with immunization but not clear (e.g. missing platelet counts) or onset of thrombocytopenia after day 10 | Platelet count fall too early (without recent heparin exposure) |
| Thrombosis or other sequelae (e.g. skin lesions) | New thrombosis; skin necrosis; post-heparin bolus acute systemic reaction | Progressive or recurrent thrombosis; erythematous skin lesions; suspected thrombosis not yet proven | None |
| Other causes for thrombocytopenia not evident | No other cause for platelet count fall is evident | Possible other cause is evident | Definite other cause is present |

Pre-test probability score: 6–8 = high; 4–5 = intermediate; 0–3 = low.
*First day of immunizing heparin exposure considered day 0; the day the platelet count begins to fall is considered the day of onset of thrombocytopenia (it generally takes 1–3 days more until an arbitrary threshold that defines thrombocytopenia is passed).

probability is high, heparin should be stopped and an alternative anticoagulant given whilst laboratory tests are performed. Heparin-induced thrombocytopenia antibodies can be measured by immunological techniques or by platelet activation assays. However, these tests may be difficult to interpret as they can be abnormal in patients who do not have clinical HIT and *vice versa*. The diagnosis, therefore, is largely a clinical one and the pre-test probability should be considered when interpreting the results of laboratory tests.

Treatment of HIT requires the immediate cessation of heparin therapy but also the use of alternative anticoagulants. Low-molecular-weight heparin is not an appropriate alternative if HIT develops during treatment with UFH because there is a significant risk of cross-reactivity. In the UK the alternative anticoagulants licensed for use in HIT are danaparoid and lepirudin. Prospective studies in patients with HIT have shown that lepirudin reduced the occurrence of new thrombotic events by more than 90% but increased bleeding risk was recorded.[11]

The introduction of warfarin should be delayed until resolution of the thrombocytopenia as it can increase the risk of microvascular thrombosis in HIT. It can then be introduced but should overlap with the alternative anticoagulant. Bleeding is uncommon in HIT and as platelet transfusions could theoretically contribute to thrombotic risk they are relatively contraindicated.

## Vena cava filters

For some patients who develop a pulmonary embolus despite anticoagulation, or related to HIT as in this situation, a vena cava filter may be appropriate. It is important to establish that anticoagulation was not subtherapeutic at the time of diagnosis. An option to consider is increasing the target International Normalized Ratio (INR). Increasing the target INR to 3.5 in patients on oral anticoagulant therapy who develop recurrent VTE with a target of 2.5 and an INR greater than 2.0 at the time of recurrent thrombosis has been suggested.[12] In the situation described in the case history above, oral anticoagulation is not appropriate given the hepatic impairment secondary to liver metastases and insertion of a vena cava filter is an option. However, in general, caval filters in cancer patients are more often associated with filter-related thrombosis.

The British Committee for Standards in Haematology has recently produced detailed guidelines on the use of vena cava filters.[13]

## Recent Developments

Patients require different warfarin dosages to achieve the target therapeutic range. This is partly explained by many environmental/acquired factors such as diet, compliance, drugs and intercurrent illness. The variability is also largely genetically determined. It is partly explained by genetic variability in the cytochrome CYP2C9 locus, the liver enzyme required for oxidative metabolism of many drugs. Two variant alleles have been associated with decreased warfarin dose requirements, more time to achieve stable dosing, a higher risk of bleeding during the initiation phase and a significantly higher bleeding rate.

However, allelic variants of CYP2C9 do not explain the large interindividual variability in the dose–anticoagulant effect of warfarin, suggesting that additional factors may contribute to this variability. Recently, a novel gene responsible, at least in part, for the activity of the vitamin K epoxide reductase (VKOR) complex, the vitamin K epoxide reductase complex subunit 1 (*VKORC1*) gene, has been identified.[14] Four different heterozygous missense mutations have been found in patients suffering from warfarin resistance.

Current anticoagulant drugs have limitations, which has fuelled the impetus to develop new drugs. These can be classified according to which steps in the coagulation process they act on and fall into four broad categories: inhibitors of initiation of coagulation, inhibitors of propagation of coagulation (fondaparinux), modulators of the protein C pathway and thrombin inhibitors (ximelagatran).

New anticoagulant drugs form the subject of a detailed review article.[15] Fondaparinux is a synthetic indirect inhibitor of activated factor X. It exerts its effect by selectively binding to antithrombin and producing a conformational change that increases the anti-Xa activity of antithrombin (an endogenous anticoagulant) approximately 300 fold. It is given once a day via the subcutaneous route and has a predictable anticoagulant response hence routine monitoring is not required. It does not bind to platelet factor 4 so HIT is unlikely. Trials have shown it is as effective and safe as LMWH for treatment of DVT.

Thrombin inhibitors prevent fibrin formation and thrombin-mediated feedback activation of coagulation factors. In North America, hirudin and argatroban are licensed for treatment of HIT.

Ximelagatran is the first orally available direct thrombin inhibitor. It has a predictable anticoagulant effect hence no monitoring is required. However, it is eliminated via the kidneys and may require dose reduction in patients with renal impairment. Efficacy has been demonstrated for thromboprophylaxis in high-risk orthopaedic surgery and treatment of VTE. Unfortunately it has caused significant increases in liver transaminases, often more than three times the upper limit of normal; whilst in the majority of cases this caused no symptoms and was reversible, one trial patient developed serious liver injury.

Dabigatran, another oral direct thrombin inhibitor, is under evaluation and to date has not been reported to cause liver dysfunction.

## Conclusion

 Venous thromboembolism is a common complication in the cancer patient and management may be complex. Low-molecular-weight heparin is the treatment of choice and the potential antineoplastic effect of LMWH confers possible additional benefit; results from further studies are awaited.

Heparin-induced thrombocytopenia is not an infrequent complication of heparin therapy. Awareness of the condition is increasing and scoring systems are now available to assess the probability of its occurrence.

Several new anticoagulants are under evaluation; oral direct thrombin inhibitors show promise. However, the precise role of these newer agents is yet to be defined and for many there is no effective reversal agent.

## Further Reading

1  Shen VS, Pollak EW. Fatal pulmonary embolism in cancer patients: is heparin prophylaxis justified? *South Med J* 1980; **73**: 841–3.

2  Rajgopal R, Bear M, Butcher MK, Shaughnessy SG. The effects of heparin and low molecular weight heparins on bone. *Thromb Res* 2008; **122**: 293–8.

3  Baglin T, Barrowcliffe T, Cohen A, Greaves M for the British Committee for Standards in Haematology. Guidelines on the use and monitoring of heparin. *Br J Haematol* 2006; **133**: 19–34.

4  Greaves M. Limitations of the laboratory monitoring of heparin therapy. *Thromb Haemost* 2002; **87**: 163–4.

5  Prandoni P. How I treat venous thromboembolism in patients with cancer. *Blood* 2005; **106**: 4027–33.

6  Altinbas M, Coskun H, Er O, *et al.* A randomized clinical trial of combination chemotherapy with and without low-molecular-weight heparin in small cell lung cancer. *J Thromb Haemost* 2004; **2**: 1266–71.

7  Kakkar AK, Levine MN, Kadizola J, *et al.* Low molecular weight heparin, therapy with dalteparin, and survival in advanced cancer: the Fragmin Advanced Malignancy Outcome Study (FAMOUS). *J Clin Oncol* 2004; **22**: 1944–8.

8  Lee AY, Levine NM, Baker RI, *et al.* Low-molecular-weight heparin versus a coumarin for the prevention of recurrent venous thromboembolism in patients with cancer. *N Engl J Med* 2003; **349**: 146–53.

9  Baglin TP, Keeling DM, Watson HG. Guidelines on oral anticoagulation (warfarin): third edition – 2005 update. *Br J Haematol* 2005; **132**: 277–85.

10 Martel N, Lee J, Wells P. Risk for heparin-induced thrombocytopenia with unfractionated and low-molecular-weight heparin thromboprophylaxis: a meta-analysis. *Blood* 2005; **106**: 2710–15.

11  Warkentin TE. Heparin-induced thrombocytopenia: pathogenesis and management. *Br J Haematol* 2003; **121**: 535–55.

12  Warkentin TE, Heddle NM. Laboratory diagnosis of immune heparin-induced thrombocytopenia. *Curr Hematol Rep* 2003; **2**: 148–57.

13  Baglin T, Brush J, Streiff M for the British Committee for Standards in Haematology. Guidelines on use of vena cava filters. *Br J Haematol* 2006; **134**: 590–95.

14  D'Andrea G, D'Ambrosio R, Di Perna P, *et al.* A polymorphism in the *VKORC1* gene is associated with an interindividual variability in the dose–anticoagulant effect of warfarin. *Blood* 2005; **105**: 645–9.

15  Bates SM, Weitz J. The status of new anticoagulants. *Br J Haematol* 2006; **134**: 3–19.

## PROBLEM

# 03  Bleeding in an intensive therapy unit patient

## Case History

 A 68-year-old man was admitted to Accident and Emergency with a 6-hour history of increasing abdominal pain and diarrhoea. He was a heavy smoker with a history of ischaemic heart disease. On examination he had a pulsatile mass present in his abdomen and no lower limb pulses. A computed tomography scan of his abdomen confirmed a leaking abdominal aortic aneurysm. Haemoglobin was 4 g/dl, white cell count $12 \times 10^9$/l, platelet count $432 \times 10^9$/l and coagulation screen was normal. Intra-operatively he lost approximately 10 litres of blood and was transfused 15 units of red cells. He also initially required large volumes of colloids to maintain his blood pressure. On the intensive therapy unit (ITU) post-operatively he was noted to be bleeding from drain sites at a rate that was higher than anticipated and was oozing from his arterial line and central venous pressure (CVP) line sites. Data from a repeat full blood count and coagulation screen were: haemoglobin 12 g/l, white cell count $16 \times 10^9$/l, platelet count $15 \times 10^9$/l, prothrombin time (PT) 22 seconds, activated partial thromboplastin time (APTT) 60 seconds, fibrinogen 0.8 g/l.

**You are asked for your advice regarding the patient's blood results. How would you manage this case?**

# Background

Major bleeding, and consequently massive transfusion (MT), is a frequent complication of surgery. Massive transfusion is defined as replacement of one blood volume within a 24-hour period, the normal adult blood volume being about 7% of ideal body weight. Massively transfused patients show evidence of defective haemostasis in a high number of cases, but the incidence varies depending on the clinical context (blunt versus penetrating trauma, elective versus emergency surgery) and according to the definition of coagulopathy (clinical findings versus laboratory test results) and to the blood products administered to the patient. The cause of coagulopathy in MT is multifactorial, secondary to haemodilution of coagulation factors and platelets, disseminated intravascular coagulation (DIC), hypothermia, acidosis and hypocalcaemia.[1]

Haemodilution occurs following volume replacement with crystalloid or colloid and transfusion of red cells, and results in a reduction in the concentrations of platelets and coagulation factors. The level of fibrinogen is reduced first, with a level of 1 g/l after 150% blood volume loss, followed by a fall of coagulation factors to 25% activity after 200% blood loss. Prolongation of the APTT and PT to 1.5 times the mean normal values is associated with an increased risk of clinical coagulopathy. A platelet count of at least $50 \times 10^9$/l occurs when about two blood volumes have been replaced by fluid or red cells.

Disseminated intravascular coagulation is an acquired syndrome secondary to the systemic activation of coagulation. It is associated with the haemostatic defects related to the excessive generation of thrombin and fibrin and the excessive consumption of platelets and coagulation factors. This results in the clinical signs of end-organ damage from microthrombi in small vessels and microvascular oozing. Disseminated intravascular coagulation can be seen in a number of situations and often complicates the management of MT. Patients at risk are those with tissue damage secondary to tissue hypoxia, hypovolaemia or extensive muscle damage. A PT and APTT that are prolonged in excess of that expected by dilution, thrombocytopenia and a fibrinogen less than 1 g/l are highly suggestive of DIC. D-dimers may also be raised but are not diagnostic of the syndrome.

Hypothermia (temperature below 35°C) impairs thrombin generation and the formation of platelet plugs and fibrin clots, and increases clot lysis.

A summary of the interplay between the various factors associated with massive blood loss and MT is shown in Figure 3.1.

## Management

In addition to addressing any surgically remediable cause of bleeding, the appropriate use of blood component therapy is indicated in correcting the coagulopathy. Close liaison is required between clinicians and laboratory staff in this regard, in order that a rational approach to treatment is adopted. Regular checks of laboratory parameters are important in order to assess the efficacy of component replacement and guide future therapy. Importantly, the measurement of fibrinogen should be performed using the Clauss method, and not derived from the PT, as this is more reliable.

It is now recognized that patients receiving a massive red cell transfusion should also receive platelets, fresh frozen plasma (FFP; as a source of coagulation factors) or cryoprecipitate (as a source of fibrinogen). There are no universally accepted guidelines for the replacement of these blood components and recommendations are largely made based on consensus opinion rather than from evidence from controlled trials. Moreover,

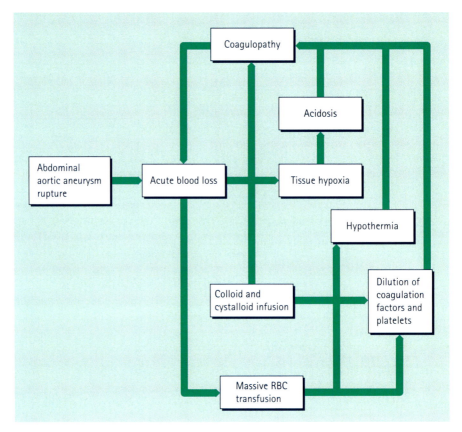

**Figure 3.1** A summary of the interplay between the various factors associated with massive blood loss and massive transfusion. RBC, red blood cell.

whether this replacement should be done prophylactically after a certain number of units of red cells or only when there is clinical or laboratory evidence of coagulopathy, as in this case, is open to some debate.

The British Committee for Standards in Haematology (BCSH) guidelines on MT advise that the platelet count should not be allowed to fall below $50 \times 10^9/l$, and that a trigger of $75 \times 10^9/l$ be observed when there is ongoing bleeding in order to provide a margin of safety.[2] The guideline from the American Society of Anesthesiology also uses $50 \times 10^9/l$ as a cut-off for platelet transfusion.[3]

The BCSH guidelines recommend that FFP (at 12–15 ml/kg) should be given after one blood volume is lost, and that the dose should be large enough to maintain coagulation factors above the critical level to ensure that the PT and APTT are less than 1.5 times the mean control level. When the fibrinogen level is critically low (<1 g/l), as in this case, it is advised that fibrinogen be replaced (two packs of pooled cryoprecipitate for an adult). Cryoprecipitate is a better source of fibrinogen than FFP and should be used.

There are data available to suggest that a minimal haematocrit (HCT) is required to achieve haemostasis. This level remains unknown, although an HCT of about 35% is often quoted. Finally, maintaining the patient in a normothermic state is also an impor-

**Table 3.1** Summary of recommendations for replacement of blood products in patients with massive bleeding

| Goal | Procedure | Comments |
|---|---|---|
| • Maintain platelets >75 × 10⁹/l | • Anticipate platelet count <50 × 10⁹/l after 2 × blood volume replacement | • Allows margin of safety to ensure platelets >50 × 10⁹/l<br>• Keep platelets >100 × 10⁹/l if multiple or CNS trauma or if platelet function abnormal |
| • Maintain PT and APTT <1.5 × mean control | • Give FFP 12–15 ml/kg (I litre or 4 units for an adult) guided by tests<br>• Anticipate need for FFP after 1–1.5 × blood volume replacement | • PT/APTT >1.5 × mean normal value correlates with increased microvascular bleeding<br>• Keep ionized Ca²⁺ >1.13 mmol/l |
| • Maintain fibrinogen >1.0 g/l | • If not corrected by FFP give cryoprecipitate (two packs of pooled cryoprecipitate for an adult) | • Cryoprecipitate rarely needed except in DIC |
| • Avoid DIC | • Treat underlying cause (shock, hypothermia, acidosis) | • Although rare, mortality is high |

APTT, activated partial thromboplastin time; CNS, central nervous system; DIC, disseminated intravascular coagulation; FFP, fresh frozen plasma; PT, prothrombin time.

tant measure in the management of the coagulopathy and in achieving haemostasis. A summary of the recommendations for blood product replacement is given in Table 3.1.

The patient continues to bleed approximately 500 ml/hour into the wound drain. He has received 2 l of FFP, four packs of pooled cryoprecipitate and four pools of platelets. He is taken back to theatre for an exploratory laparotomy, but no obvious bleeding point is identified. His coagulation profile is now normal and his platelet count is 76 × 10⁹/l.

**What would you advise regarding the management of the bleeding?**

## Background

The patient has 'normal' haemostasis based on the laboratory parameters but continues to bleed, with no surgically correctable cause found. This refractory coagulopathic bleeding is not uncommon, with approximately 50% of the mortality in patients with traumatic bleeding attributed to it. The limitations of conventional blood products emphasize the need for additional haemostatic agents. Antifibrinolytic agents such as aprotinin, tranexamic acid and ε-aminocaproic acid have been shown to reduce surgical blood loss. In addition, 1-deamino-8-D-arginine vasopressin (DDAVP) can improve haemostasis in patients with uraemia and hepatic failure. Finally, fibrin glue has been used effectively when applied directly to a bleeding point. However, none of these agents has been shown to be effective in stopping coagulopathic bleeding. Rather, they have been shown to be most effective at prevention of rebleeding.

Recombinant factor VIIa (rFVIIa) was first used in the 1980s as a haemostatic agent. Since then it has been licensed for use in haemophilic patients with inhibitors to coagulation factors VIII or IX and in patients with platelet function defects. However, more recently its off-license use has been extended to include treatment of massive bleeding in a number of different clinical situations. Based on the current cell-based model of

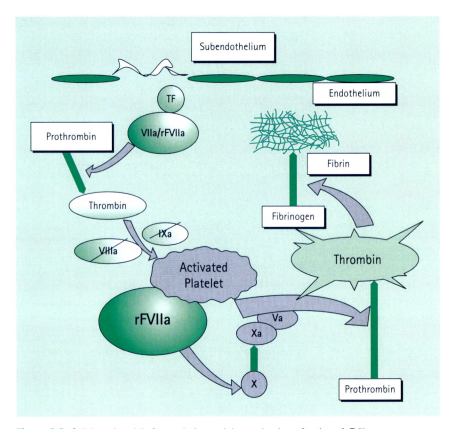

**Figure 3.2** Cell-based model of coagulation and the mechanism of action of rFVIIa.

coagulation,[4] rFVIIa is thought to act locally at the site of tissue injury rather than systemically. It binds to exposed tissue factor (TF), and the rFVIIa–TF complex initiates coagulation by activating factor X (FX) and factor IX (FIX). Factor Xa then forms a complex with its cofactor factor V (FV) on the surface of activated platelets. This is sufficient to activate prothrombin and produce a small amount of thrombin. This is insufficient to convert fibrinogen to a fibrin clot, but further accelerates the coagulation cascade by activating FV, factor VIII (FVIII), factor XI (FXI) and additional platelets. This results in production of a large amount of thrombin, the so-called 'thrombin burst', which changes soluble fibrinogen into insoluble fibrin. Administration of pharmacological doses of rFVIIa causes faster and higher thrombin generation. It also binds to the phospholipid membrane of activated platelets and activates FX and FIX in a TF-independent manner, which further accelerates the coagulation process. This process is illustrated in Figure 3.2.

There has been an increasing number of case reports and case series on the use of rFVIIa in various clinical situations since the first report of its use in a trauma patient in 1999.[5] However, evidence from controlled trials is lacking. In one trial, 36 patients underwent abdominal prostatectomy and were randomized to a single injection of rFVIIa (20 or 40 µg/kg) or placebo during the operation.[6] Administration of 40 µg/kg of rFVIIa at the beginning of the operation resulted in a 50% reduction of blood loss compared to placebo, and reduced the need for blood transfusion. Another controlled trial of 301 patients with blunt or penetrating trauma showed that red cell transfusion was reduced in the rFVIIa arm, and that there was a trend towards lower mortality rates when rFVIIa was used.[7] Despite this, however, there is conflicting evidence to support the use of rFVIIa as a 'last-ditch' treatment for massive haemorrhage. A recent review of the use of rFVIIa for treatment of severe bleeding concluded that it appeared to be relatively safe with 1%–2% incidence of thrombotic complications based on published trials.[8]

### Management with recombinant factor VIIa

The BCSH guidelines on MT suggest that, until more evidence is available from controlled trials, rFVIIa should be considered for use where there is blood loss of >300 ml/hr.[2] Moreover, it should only be used when there is no evidence of heparin or warfarin effect, where surgical control of bleeding has been explored and when adequate replacement of coagulation factors (FFP, cryoprecipitate and platelets) and correction of acidosis have been achieved. The guidelines also recommend that local policies and guidelines should be in place to aid decisions regarding treatment with rFVIIa.

There is no agreed dosage, schedule or timing for the administration of rFVIIa in the massively bleeding patient. In the UK, the licensed dose for patients with haemophilia and inhibitors is 90 µg/kg. The same dose has been used in patients with massive bleeding. However, guidelines produced by the Israeli Multidisciplinary rFVIIa Task Force suggest that the dose may need to be higher (100–140 µg/kg).[9] A repeat dose of 100 µg/kg should be administered if bleeding persists beyond 15–20 minutes after the initial dose. A third dose should only be given after coagulation has been rechecked and corrected with blood products or empirical treatment given. Currently there are no laboratory methods for monitoring efficacy of rFVIIa. Response should be judged based on clinical response, although techniques such as thromboelastography and thrombin generation measurements could be used as objective measures of response in the future.

# Recent Developments

The use of rFVIIa in non-haemophiliac patients anticipated to be at risk of major bleeding (prophylactic) or who have uncontrolled bleeding (therapeutic) has been a subject for debate. Review of randomized controlled trial (RCT) evidence for effectiveness of rFVIIa in these situations has been undertaken.[10] In particular, the effect of rFVIIa on blood loss and transfusion requirement was analysed. A significant reduction in transfusion requirements and/or blood loss in the rFVIIa-treated groups were recorded, but has not been confirmed in large randomised trials. Use in intracranial haemorrhage showed both bleed progression and mortality were reduced although preliminary results from a subsequent phase III trial have found no outcome benefit. The thromboembolic adverse event incidence in subjects who received rFVIIa is of concern and occurred despite exclusion criterion of patients with a history of previous thromboembolic or vasoocclusive disease. Further evidence is needed from appropriately designed clinical trials to better assess the optimal dose, efficacy and the safety of rFVIIa in critical bleeding conditions.

## Conclusion

Bleeding in the ITU patient is a common problem and can be seen in a number of different clinical situations. The case presented here is of a patient undergoing an emergency aortic aneurysm repair. It highlights the importance of systematic review of the patient and of looking for surgically correctable causes and deranged coagulation profiles that can be reversed by the administration of fractionated blood components. Only after these avenues have been explored should the use of newer haemostatic agents, which have yet to prove their efficacy in this area, be considered.

## Further Reading

1 Hardy J, de Moerloose P, Samama M. Massive transfusion and coagulopathy: pathophysiology and implications for clinical management. *Can J Anaesth* 2004; **51**: 293–310.

2 Stainsby D, MacLennan S, Thomas D, Isaac J, Hamilton PJ. Guidelines on the management of massive blood loss. *Br J Haematol* 2006; **135**: 634–41.

3 Practice guidelines for blood component therapy: a report by the American Society of Anesthesiologists Task Force on Blood Component Therapy. *Anesthesiology* 1996; **84**: 732–47.

4 Hoffman M. A cell-based model of coagulation and the role of factor VIIa. *Blood Rev* 2003; **17(Suppl 1)**: s1–s5.

5 Kenet G, Walden R, Eldad A, Martinowitz U. Treatment of traumatic bleeding with recombinant factor VIIa. *Lancet* 1999; **354**: 1879.

6 Friederich P, Henny CP, Messelink EJ, *et al*. Effect of recombinant activated factor VII on perioperative blood loss in patients undergoing retropubic prostatectomy: a double-blind placebo-controlled randomised trial. *Lancet* 2003; **361**: 201–5.

7 Boffard K, Warren B, Iau P, *et al*. Decreased transfusion utilization and improved outcome associated with the use of recombinant factor VIIa as an adjunct in trauma. *J Trauma* 2004; **57**: 451.

8 Levi M, Peters M, Buller HR. Efficacy and safety of recombinant factor VIIa for treatment of severe bleeding: a systematic review. *Crit Care Med* 2005; **33**: 883–90.

9 Martinowitz U, Michaelson M. Guidelines for the use of recombinant activated factor VII (rFVIIa) in uncontrolled bleeding: a report by the Israeli Multidisciplinary rFVIIa Task Force. *J Thromb Haemost* 2005; **3**: 640–48.

10 Johansson PI. Off-label use of recombinant factor VIIa for treatment of haemorrhage: results from randomized clinical trials. *Vox Sang* 2008; **95**: 1–7.

# 04  Investigation of easy bruising

## Case History

A 28-year-old woman is referred by her General Practitioner as she is complaining of easy bruising and menorrhagia.

**What further information would you like?**

## Background

### Initial management

A thorough, detailed history of the bleeding is vital in the assessment of patients with potential haemostatic defects, and it will impact on the extent of investigation.

The duration of bleeding/bruising is important when considering whether the patient is likely to have a congenital or acquired haemostatic disorder. Bleeding since childhood, such as menorrhagia since menarche, would usually suggest a congenital disorder; however, mild congenital disorders of coagulation may present in adult life.[1] A family history of abnormal bleeding clearly would also support the presence of a congenital defect.

It is useful to establish the details of bruising, in particular whether it is spontaneous, occurs after minimal trauma or after surgery, and its extent.

Tonsillectomy and dental extraction in particular pose significant haemostatic challenges and if these have not been associated with significant bleeding, a congenital disorder of haemostasis is much less likely.

Bleeding or bruising on multiple occasions and from different sites merits more extensive investigation as this suggests a systemic haemostatic defect. Repeatedly bleeding from one site, such as epistaxis from the same nostril, suggests a structural abnormality.

Mucocutaneous bleeding (epistaxis, bruising, menorrhagia, gastrointestinal bleeding) as in this case suggests a disorder of platelet function.

Coagulation factor deficiencies are more likely to be associated with haemarthrosis, muscle haematoma and post-operative bleeding.

Although menorrhagia is a common gynaecological symptom, a specific cause is identified in less than 50% of affected women.[2] Studies have shown that bleeding disorders are found in a substantial proportion of women with menorrhagia and a normal pelvis examination. Inherited bleeding disorders have been diagnosed in 17% of such patients, with von Willebrand's disease being the most common abnormality.[2]

Systemic illness, in particular uraemia and liver disease, may cause abnormalities of haemostasis (Table 4.1).

A detailed drug history is clearly relevant; aspirin and non-steroidal anti-inflammatory agents are common culprits causing platelet function defects, but many drugs are implicated (Table 4.2).

**Table 4.1 Causes of platelet disorders**

| Congenital | Acquired |
| --- | --- |
| von Willebrand's disease | Liver disease |
| Abnormality of platelet membrane glycoprotein (e.g. Bernard–Soulier syndrome, Glanzmann thrombasthenia) | Uraemia |
| Abnormality of platelet granules (e.g. storage pool disorder, grey platelet syndrome) | Myeloma/monoclonal gammopathy of uncertain significance |
| Abnormalities of signal transduction and secretion (e.g. defects in arachidonic acid metabolism – cyclooxygenase deficiency) | Myeloproliferative disorders |
| | Leukaemia/myelodysplasia |
| | Sepsis |
| | Cardiopulmonary bypass |
| | Drugs |

**Table 4.2 Drugs and other agents known to interfere with platelet function**

| |
| --- |
| Aspirin |
| Non-steroidal anti-inflammatory agents |
| Antibiotics (penicillins, cephalosporins) |
| Cardiovascular drugs (propranolol, nifedipine, isosorbide mononitrate) |
| Volume expanders (dextrans) |
| Psychotropic drugs (amitriptyline, chlorpromazine, haloperidol) |
| Local anaesthetic |
| Antihistamines |
| Radiographic contrast agents |
| Alcohol |
| Foods (cumin, turmeric, fish oils) |

Of the drugs listed, only aspirin has been demonstrated to cause a significant increase in bleeding although the other drugs can affect tests of platelet function.

Clinical examination should focus on any bleeding, bruising or evidence of underlying systemic illness, particularly liver disease or a primary haematological disorder.

This lady has significant menorrhagia and marked bruising. She is not taking any medication and has no family history of abnormal bleeding, although her mother died in her thirties.

**How would you investigate her?**

## Investigation strategy

The patient's history is suggestive of a platelet disorder or von Willebrand's disease. Von Willebrand factor (VWF) is a plasma protein that mediates platelet adhesion to the subendothelium, mediates platelet aggregation and serves as a transport protein for factor VIII.

When vessel wall damage occurs, platelets undergo many responses including adhesion, release reactions, aggregation, exposure of a procoagulant surface, formation of microparticles and clot retraction. These changes lead to rapid formation of a haemostatic plug at the site of damage, which prevents blood loss. Defects in any of these functions and/or platelet number usually cause impaired haemostasis and increased risk of bleeding.

Baseline investigations should include a full blood count to look for thrombocytopenia and a blood film. The blood film is important to look for evidence of a primary haematological disorder such as myelodysplasia, to assess platelet morphology and to show any abnormalities suggestive of hepatic or renal dysfunction.

A basic coagulation screen should be performed; this should include measurements of the prothrombin time, activated partial thromboplastin time and fibrinogen.

If her history was not particularly suggestive of a bleeding tendency, then the above investigations are probably sufficient.

However, her history is convincing despite these initial tests being normal, hence she requires further investigation. The next step would be to screen her for von Willebrand's disease and assess her platelet function using a platelet function analyser (PFA-100® system). Depending on the results she may require further assessment of her platelet function by performing platelet aggregometry, platelet glycoprotein analysis and platelet nucleotide analysis (Figure 4.1).

# Recent Developments

### The role of the platelet function analyser

The platelet function analyser (PFA) was developed in the mid-1990s to assess primary haemostasis *in vitro* and provide a simple global measure of high-shear platelet function. It works by aspirating citrated blood from the sample reservoir through a capillary tube. The blood sample is applied to a collagen-coated membrane containing a 150 µm aperture in the presence of epinephrine or adenosine diphosphate (ADP). The membrane is contained in disposable cartridges. Blood flow through the aperture is monitored. The platelets start to adhere and aggregate resulting in occlusion of the aperture between 1 and 3 minutes from the start of the test. The time taken for occlusion of the aperture (closure time) is recorded. The flow rate drops as platelets form a haemostatic plug within the aperture.

The PFA is a quick, relatively straightforward test and hence does not require detailed specialist training of staff to use it. It has a high negative predictive value and is useful as a screening tool. The PFA can be used to exclude von Willebrand's disease and severe congenital platelet defects, particularly Bernard–Soulier syndrome and Glanzmann thrombasthenia.

The PFA is now thought to be superior (more sensitive) to the bleeding time, which has limitations and may be insensitive to many mild platelet defects. The bleeding time does not necessarily correlate with or predict bleeding tendency.[3]

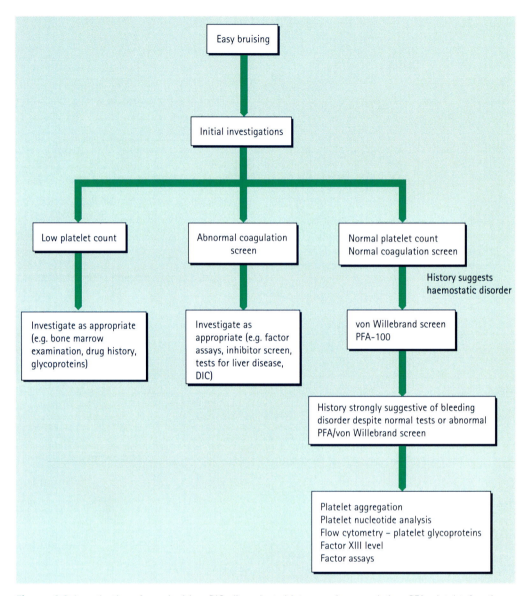

**Figure 4.1** Investigation of easy bruising. DIC, disseminated intravascular coagulation; PFA, platelet function analyser.

However, false-negative PFA results may occur in type 1 von Willebrand's disease and storage pool disorders. Results are also sensitive to acquired variables including diet and drugs and it is important to repeat the test on separate occasions.[4]

The PFA is not a diagnostic test nor is an abnormal result specific to any disorder. The results require interpretation in conjunction with results of baseline coagulation studies, a von Willebrand screen and a full blood count. If the PFA produces a normal result despite strong clinical suspicion of a bleeding disorder then further investigation is required. This would include platelet glycoprotein analysis by flow cytometry, platelet nucleotide analysis and platelet aggregometry. The PFA results are affected by thrombocytopenia and haematocrit. A platelet count below $80 \times 10^9/l$ and haematocrit below 30% will cause prolonged closure times.

The potential clinical applications for the PFA are broad. It may be used as a screening tool and can replace bleeding time given that it is more sensitive and reliable. It is also suitable for use in monitoring the effects of therapy such as DDAVP (1-deamino-8-D-arginine vasopressin [synthetic desmopressin]) in von Willebrand's disease.[5] Moreover, it has a role in monitoring the antiplatelet effect of aspirin therapy but is insensitive to the effects of clopidogrel. Initial studies for screening women with menorrhagia have looked promising but larger studies are required before this could be routinely recommended. Other potential applications include monitoring the quality control of platelet concentrates, screening platelet donors and prediction of surgical bleeding.

## Conclusion

Investigation of the patient with easy bruising or abnormal bleeding requires a structured approach working through diagnostic tests in a logical, stepwise order.

Emphasis on the importance of taking a detailed and thorough bleeding history cannot be stressed more. It is important to continue to investigate the patient despite normal initial investigations if the history is highly suggestive of a haemostatic defect. The PFA is superior to the bleeding time and is a promising screening tool for investigation of platelet disorders, although it is not 100% sensitive for all platelet disorders. Additional clinical applications for the PFA are under development.

## Further Reading

1   Khair K, Liesner R. Bruising and bleeding in infants and children – a practical approach. *Br J Haematol* 2006; **133**: 221–31.

2   Kadir RA, Economides DL, Sabin CA, Owens D, Lee CA. Frequency of inherited bleeding disorders in women with menorrhagia. *Lancet* 1998; **351**: 485–9.

3   Harrison P. The role of PFA-100 testing in the investigation and management of haemostatic defects in children and adults. *Br J Haematol* 2005; **130**: 3–10.

4   Cattaneo M. Are the bleeding time and PFA-100 useful in the initial screening of patients with mucocutaneous bleedings of hereditary nature? *J Thromb Haemost* 2004; **2**: 890–91.

5   Harrison P. Platelet function analysis. *Blood Rev* 2005; **19**: 111–23.

# 05 Inherited disorders of coagulation

## Case History

A ten-year-old boy presents with a haemarthrosis. A diagnosis of haemophilia A is suspected.

**How common are the inherited disorders of coagulation and how does the clinical phenotype vary?**

## Background

Inherited deficiencies may occur in any of the coagulation factors. However, the commonest inherited bleeding disorder is von Willebrand's disease, which is reported to affect as many as 1% of the general population. This is usually due to a quantitative deficiency in von Willebrand factor but may be due to a qualitative defect. This is usually a clinically mild bleeding disorder producing mucosal bleeding. Menorrhagia may be problematic and a significant number (17%) of women with menorrhagia and no primary gynaecological pathology have an undiagnosed bleeding disorder, with von Willebrand's disease being the most frequent.[1] The next most common disorder is haemophilia A, the deficiency of factor VIII (FVIII), followed by haemophilia B (deficiency of factor IX). The remaining inherited coagulation deficiencies are rare, although many exhibit autosomal recessive inheritance and thus are more prominent in communities where consanguinity occurs. The features of these rare inherited coagulation factor deficiencies are summarized in Table 5.1.[2]

### What is the optimum management of a patient with newly diagnosed haemophilia A?

### Background

Severe haemophilia is characterized by spontaneous bleeding into joints and muscles. If inadequately treated, the repeated bleeding causes synovial hypertrophy, which encourages recurrent bleeding, producing a 'target joint' and ultimately the development of a painful and destructive arthropathy. This particularly tends to affect the large hinge joints (knees, ankles and elbows). It is unclear why joints and muscles are the predominant sites of bleeding.

With advances in the management of haemophilia, in particular the development of safe and effective therapy, those affected can now look forward to a relatively normal life expectancy.[3] In the past, the complications of haemophilia, such as transfusion-transmitted infections and the development of antibodies rendering treatment ineffective, meant that many of these individuals died young.

**Table 5.1** Rare inherited coagulation factor deficiencies (adapted from [1])

| Factor deficiency | Prevalence | Clinical phenotype | Screening coagulation tests | Treatment |
|---|---|---|---|---|
| Fibrinogen (factor I) | 1 in 1 000 000 | Variable, spontaneous bleeding, umbilical and mucosal and ICH | Prolonged PT, APTT, TT | Personal and family history of bleeding important. Virally inactivated concentrate not licensed in Europe. Cryoprecipitate for emergencies – not virally inactivated. Aim for level of 1 g/l |
| Prothrombin (factor II) | 1 in 2 000 000 (rarest) | Hypoprothrombinaemia (type 1); dysprothrombinaemia (type 2); mucosal and soft tissue bleeding, haemarthrosis | Usually prolonged PT and APTT | No specific concentrates. Prothrombin-complex concentrates treatment of choice; can use virally inactivated FFP. Levels 20–30 IU haemostatic |
| Factor V | 1 in 1 000 000 homozygote | Moderately severe bleeding disorder – bruising and mucous membrane, haemarthrosis and muscle bleeds less common | Prolonged PT and APTT, exclude combined FV and FVIII deficiency | No concentrate available. Virally inactivated FFP. Minimum haemostatic level 15 U/dl |
| Combined FV and FVIII deficiency | 1 in 1 000 000 | Easy bruising and epistaxis, post-operative bleeding | Prolonged PT and disproportionately prolonged APTT | Treat spontaneous bleeding with FFP and FVIII concentrate – aim for recombinant FVIII 30–50 U/dl depending on severity and 25 U/dl factor V |
| Factor VII deficiency | 1 in 300 000–1 in 500 000 for severe deficiency | Bleeding spectrum variable mucous membrane, CNS bleed if severe | Prolonged PT, normal APTT | FVII concentrates, FFP if no alternative, prothrombin-complex concentrates, tranexamic acid. Levels 10–15 U/dl haemostatic |
| Factor X deficiency | I in 1 000 000 homozygous; heterozygous 1 in 500 but usually asymptomatic | Significant bleeding if severe, usually mucosal | Prolonged PT and APTT | Tranexamic acid, virally inactivated FFP, prothrombin-complex concentrates |
| Deficiency of vitamin K–dependent factors | <20 kindreds worldwide | Wide variation in phenotype – ICH, haemarthrosis, soft tissue/gastrointestinal tract bleeds | Prolonged PT and APTT | Vitamin K, FFP or prothrombin-complex concentrate if no response |
| Factor XI | 1 in 1 000 000; Ashkenazi Jews 8% heterozygote frequency | Bleeding manifestations unpredictable, spontaneous haemorrhage rare, bleeding not related to FXI level; most have few problems | Prolonged APTT | Tranexamic acid. FXI concentrates on named-patient basis – concerns regarding thrombotic potential: levels not to exceed 70 U/dl |
| Factor XIII | I in 1 000 000 | Bleeding depends on level. Umbilical stump bleeding, ICH, haematoma, haemarthrosis | Normal PT, APTT, abnormal clot solubility test, FXIII levels | Prophylactic factor concentrate, as high ICH risk in severe deficiency; long half-life given 4–6-weekly. Cryoprecipitate inferior |

APTT, activated partial thromboplastin time; CNS, central nervous system; FFP, fresh frozen plasma; ICH, intracranial haemorrhage; PT, prothrombin time; TT, thrombin time.

Haemophilia A is an X-linked recessive disorder; it affects 1 in 5000 worldwide and one-third of affected individuals have no previous family history. The condition is caused by many different genetic defects, inversion of intron 22 being the commonest. The disorder is classified as mild, moderate or severe depending on the FVIII level in the blood (Table 5.2). Factor VIII is a complex plasma glycoprotein that is synthesized mainly by the liver. It has a half-life of approximately 12 hours and circulates in plasma bound to von Willebrand factor, which serves to protect FVIII from degradation and concentrate it

| Table 5.2 Classification of haemophilia | | |
| --- | --- | --- |
| Factor level | Severity | Clinical features |
| >0.05–0.40 IU/ml (5%–40% of normal) | Mild | No spontaneous bleeds, occurs after surgery/trauma |
| 0.01–0.05 IU/ml (1%–5% of normal) | Moderate | Joint and muscle bleeding following minor injury, after trauma/surgery |
| <0.01 IU/ml (<1% of normal) | Severe | Spontaneous bleeding and after surgery/trauma |

at sites of vascular damage. The bleeding occurs because of failure of secondary haemostasis; that is, failure to stabilize the platelet plug with fibrin as a result of reduced thrombin generation.

The FVIII blood level is predictive of bleeding risk, and hence treatment strategy, as illustrated in Table 5.2. The FVIII level does not alter significantly with age in haemophilia A. However, coinheritance of thrombophilic defects such as factor V Leiden can lessen bleeding manifestations.

Usually, children with severe haemophilia are born uneventfully by vaginal delivery. The risk of intracranial bleeding in neonates is 1%–4%, which predominantly occurs in the first week of life.

## Management

If there is a family history that suggests a baby may be affected by haemophilia, close collaboration between the haematologist, obstetrician and paediatrician is vital. Vacuum extraction, forceps, scalp-blood sampling and intramuscular injections should all be avoided. The majority of children with haemophilia do not develop joint/muscle bleeds until they learn to crawl or walk but they may bleed from other sites (e.g. easy bruising) earlier. This can lead to the suspicion of non-accidental injury. Moderate haemophilia is usually diagnosed by the time the affected child reaches school age. However, mild haemophilia may not present until adulthood, with excessive bleeding following injury or surgery.

Newly diagnosed haemophiliacs need to be cared for within the setting of a comprehensive care centre or in a haemophilia centre allied to a regional comprehensive care centre to ensure access to appropriate haematological expertise in terms of diagnosis, treatment, management of complications and links with necessary specialists. The specialist services provided are detailed in Figure 5.1.

A national register to record patients with bleeding disorders registered at haemophilia centres in the UK has been in operation since the late 1960s. There are approximately 5000 individuals with haemophilia A registered.

The UK Haemophilia Centre Doctors' Organisation is a national body that aims to provide standardized and optimum care for patients across the UK and continuous development of guidelines for their management. There is a national network of approximately 22 comprehensive care centres and 80 haemophilia centres.[4]

A study in the USA has shown that leaving the comprehensive care environment was associated with a 70% higher mortality risk. This was particularly true in patients who had residual complications resulting from earlier forms of treatment.

When haemophilia is diagnosed it is important to take a detailed family history to be able to construct an accurate pedigree for counselling of other family members at risk of

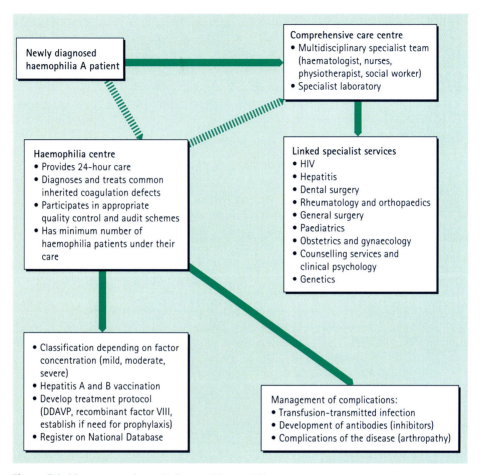

**Figure 5.1** Management of a newly diagnosed haemophiliac.

being affected or of being a carrier. For example, daughters of a haemophiliac will all carry the abnormal X chromosome making them obligate carriers.

The aim of treatment for haemophilia is to raise the concentration of FVIII sufficiently to prevent spontaneous and traumatic bleeds. In patients with mild haemophilia if treatment is required, for example to allow surgery, desmopressin (a synthetic analogue of antidiuretic hormone) is usually effective. This releases subendothelial stores of von Willebrand factor and is given via the intravenous or subcutaneous route.

Patients with moderate haemophilia do not usually have spontaneous joint bleeds hence rarely suffer long-term joint damage. Should they require treatment, they need to receive FVIII concentrates.

Patients with severe haemophilia require intravenous infusions of FVIII concentrates. Many patients are on home-therapy programmes where the FVIII is self-administered or given by a family member such as a parent.

Bleeds can be treated as they occur or treatment can be given regularly to prevent bleeds occurring (prophylaxis). Prophylactic therapy aims to abolish spontaneous joint bleeds by giving regular treatment three times a week.

In the 1970s, plasma-derived factor concentrates became available. Developments in the manufacturing led to production of high-purity concentrates, and viral-inactivation stages were introduced in the late 1980s. In 1992, recombinant FVIII concentrates were developed. The third-generation products that are now available are free from animal and human proteins and are the treatment of choice.

Today, severe haemophiliacs treated with prophylactic therapy can expect to lead a relatively normal life with few restrictions.

## Complications

Transfusion-transmitted infection from hepatitis B and C in the early plasma-derived concentrates has been recognized since the late 1970s, and infection from human immunodeficiency virus (HIV) since 1981. Hepatitis B and C viruses and HIV are destroyed by viral-inactivation steps but risks of transmission of the non-enveloped viruses (hepatitis A and parvovirus) have not been completely eliminated. It is therefore recommended that patients with inherited coagulation disorders are vaccinated against hepatitis A and B. Recently, concern has been expressed that variant Creutzfeldt–Jakob disease may be transmitted by plasma-derived concentrates; however, to date there is no evidence of such transmission.

Inhibitors are allo-antibodies to FVIII and are a serious complication of treatment with FVIII concentrates that predominantly affects severe haemophiliacs and occurs in 30%–50% of haemophilia A patients. The risk is at its highest during the first 20–100 treatments and occurs with both recombinant and plasma-derived products. Inhibitor development is related to the type of genetic mutation present, being more common in those with large deletions or inversion of intron 22. Management is complex and depends on characteristics of the inhibitors, such as titre. Options for acute bleeding events include activated prothrombin-complex concentrates, which aim to bypass factor VIII activity, or recombinant activated factor VII. Immune-tolerance regimens which use high doses of FVIII concentrates, sometimes in conjunction with immunosuppression, are used to try and eradicate inhibitors in the longer term. However, inhibitors may be transient and not all require treatment.

# Recent Developments

### Gene therapy

Haemophilia is a potential target for a gene therapy, given that only a small increase in FVIII concentration produces a significant reduction in bleeding risk. Successes in both mouse and dog models have been reported and there have now been six small clinical trials of gene transfer in haemophilia. However, no study has conclusively shown that adequate concentrations of FVIII can be reliably obtained, although no significant safety concerns have been raised. New strategies are being explored using novel viral vectors (including adeno-associated virus vectors) and transient periods of immunosuppression to reduce the host immune response to the vector and transgene product.[5]

However, haemophilia is no longer regarded as a life-threatening condition and recombinant factor concentrates are safe and effective. This should not be forgotten when considering the potential risks of gene therapy such as insertional mutagenesis, particularly since a child treated with a retroviral vector was reported to subsequently develop a haematological malignancy.

### Long-acting factor VIII preparations

While a genetic cure is awaited, perhaps through gene therapy, the question is whether innovations in drug delivery or recombinant technology will be able to overcome the barriers of cost, compliance and the need for central venous access devices necessary for effective prophylaxis. Non-invasive methods of delivery or even strategies to extend the functional half-life of FVIII could have a significant impact.

Strategies that have been successful for other therapeutic proteins are now being applied to FVIII. These include modifications such as the addition of polyethylene glycol (PEG) polymers and polysialic acids (PSA) and alternative formulation with PEG-modified liposomes.[6]

Polyethylene glycolylation of FVIII would seem to be a natural progression for the advancement of haemophilia therapeutics. The main disadvantage of PEGylated protein formulations is that an improved pharmacokinetic profile may be accompanied by decreased specific activity, although this could be compensated by a marked improvement in pharmacokinetic properties. The plasma half-life of FVIII is already extended from 2 to 12 hours through its interaction with von Willebrand factor; PEGylation of FVIII risks interfering with von Willebrand factor–FVIII affinity and compromising its plasma half-life. There is also concern as to the ultimate clearance mechanism for PEG and whether it may accumulate, particularly as there would be lifelong exposure to significant amounts of PEG. The potential adverse effects of this are unknown.

The strong hydrophilicity of the PSA could theoretically cause a 'watery cloud' to form around the therapeutic molecule protecting it from proteolytic enzymes. Moreover, PSA are biodegradable giving them an advantage over PEGylation when applied to a therapeutic protein that will be delivered in large doses and over an extended period of time. Polysialylation holds promise for extending the half-life of FVIII without compromising its functional activity. It may even reduce the immunogenicity of FVIII or protect it from neutralizing antibodies in patients with inhibitors. It is unclear whether polysialylated FVIII can retain von Willebrand factor affinity and still be effectively activated by thrombin.

In addition, targeted modifications of the FVIII protein may increase the duration of its cofactor activity and reduce its clearance. These stabilized forms of activated FVIII hold promise for the future.

# Conclusion

### Global advances

The outlook for people with severe haemophilia differs substantially between countries. A dramatic improvement on the quality of life and life expectancy is gained by national haemophilia programmes. The World Federation of Hemophilia has shown that survival is increased by the development of treatment centres and the use of replacement therapy.[7]

The World Federation of Hemophilia has also developed a network of training centres and a twinning programme between centres in more-developed countries and partners in less-developed countries to promote sharing of expertise. The aim is to help treatment centres in poorer countries improve haemophilia care. The programme began in 1994 and there are more than 30 partnerships at present.

## Further Reading

1 Kadir RA, Economides DL, Sabin CA, Owens D, Lee CA. Frequency of inherited bleeding disorders in women with menorrhagia. *Lancet* 1998; **351**: 485–9.

2 Bolton-Maggs PHB, Perry DJ, Chalmers EA, *et al.* The rare coagulation disorders – review with guidelines for management from the United Kingdom Haemophilia Centre Doctors' Organisation. *Haemophilia* 2004; **10**: 593–628.

3 Soucie JM, Nuss R, Evatt B, *et al.* Mortality among males with hemophilia: relations with source of medical care. *Blood* 2000; **96**: 437–42.

4 The Haemophilia Alliance. A national service specification for haemophilia and other inherited bleeding disorders, 2006. www.haemophiliaalliance.org.uk/

5 Lillicrap D, VandenDriessche T, High K. Cellular and genetic therapies for haemophilia. *Haemophilia* 2006; **12(Suppl 3)**: 36–41.

6 Saenko EL, Pipe SW. Strategies towards a longer acting factor VIII. *Haemophilia* 2006; **12(Suppl 3)**: 42–51.

7 Bolton-Maggs PHB, Pasi KJ. Haemophilias A and B. *Lancet* 2003; **361**: 1801–9.

**PROBLEM**

# 06 Thrombophilia

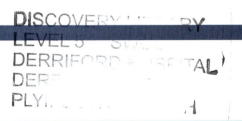

## Case History

A 44-year-old man develops a lower limb deep vein thrombosis with no apparent risk factors.

**Should he be investigated for thrombophilia?**

## Background

The British Committee for Standards in Haematology (1990) defines thrombophilia as 'disorders of the haemostatic mechanisms which are likely to predispose to thrombosis'. This definition encompasses acquired and inherited thrombophilia. Acquired thrombophilic states include surgery, nephrotic syndrome, inflammatory disorders, hormone use and pregnancy. Inherited thrombophilia is a genetically determined tendency to thrombosis.

This definition is now widely used but has disadvantages. First, many individuals who carry these defects never have a thrombotic event. Secondly, despite an increasing num-

| Table 6.1 Thrombophilic defects | | |
|---|---|---|
| **Inherited** | **Acquired – environmental** | **Combined** |
| Antithrombin deficiency | Lupus anticoagulant | Elevated factor VIII level |
| Protein C deficiency | Dysfibrinogenaemia | Elevated factor XI level |
| Protein S deficiency | | Elevated factor IX level |
| Prothrombin gene mutation | | |
| Factor V Leiden mutation | | |
| Dysfibrinogenaemia | | |

ber of thrombophilic risk factors that can be tested for, at least 50% of patients presenting with a history of thrombosis do not have an identifiable laboratory defect.[1]

A more clinically useful definition of thrombophilia is used in North America where the term is used to describe patients who have developed venous thrombosis either spontaneously or of a severity out of proportion to any recognized stimulus, patients who have recurrent venous thrombotic events and patients who develop venous thrombosis at an early age.

Thrombophilia screening includes measurement of the natural anticoagulants (protein C, protein S, antithrombin) and the common mutations, as shown in Table 6.1.

## Inherited thrombophilic defects

A small number of genetic variants are independent risk factors for venous thromboembolism (VTE). These include mutations in the genes encoding the natural anticoagulants – antithrombin, protein C and protein S – and the clotting factors fibrinogen, prothrombin and factor V. Levels fluctuate and hence the finding of a low level of a natural anticoagulant on a single occasion is not diagnostic of primary deficiency and *vice versa*. There are no guidelines on the number of times that measurements should be repeated or on the extent of family testing required to confirm or exclude deficiencies in these anticoagulant proteins.

### Activated protein C resistance and factor V Leiden

Factor V Leiden is the most common cause of inherited activated protein C (APC) resistance, defined as an impaired plasma anticoagulant response to APC added *in vitro*.

This impaired response is caused by a point mutation in the gene for clotting factor V (G1691A) rendering the protein more resistant to degradation. However, APC resistance may be acquired by those using an oestrogen-containing contraceptive pill, by pregnancy and by hormone replacement therapy. The effect is more marked with third-generation compared with second-generation oral contraceptives.

The most commonly used test system for APC resistance is the activated partial thromboplastin time (APTT). Samples are tested with and without added APC and the resultant clotting times are expressed as a ratio (APC sensitivity ratio). Factor V Leiden is the commonest thrombophilic defect in Northern Europe with a reported prevalence of 2%–5%. Heterozygous carriers have a three- to eightfold increased risk of venous thrombosis; homozygotes have an 80-fold increased risk.

## Protein C deficiency

Protein C is a vitamin K-dependent protein that is synthesized in the liver. It is an inhibitor of coagulation. It exerts its effect by degrading activated factor V and factor VIII, with protein S working as a cofactor.

Reduced protein C activity is seen in patients with disseminated intravascular coagulation, in those receiving coumarins and in liver disease. Protein C deficiency confers between a 10- and 15-fold relative risk of VTE.

## Protein S deficiency

Protein S is also a vitamin K-dependent protein, which functions as a cofactor for APC. The interaction between protein C and protein S is illustrated in Figure 6.1. Quantitative and qualitative defects in protein S have been identified.

Protein S levels fall progressively during pregnancy. They are also lowered to a lesser extent by the oral contraceptive pill, hormone replacement therapy, coumarins, disseminated intravascular coagulation and liver disease.

The prevalence of protein S deficiency in the general population remains unknown.

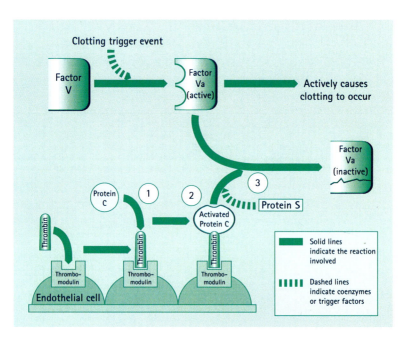

**Figure 6.1** The protein C–protein S system.

## Antithrombin deficiency

Antithrombin is synthesized by the liver. In addition to inhibiting thrombin, it also inhibits the activated clotting factors IXa, Xa, XIa, XIIa and tissue factor–bound factor VIIa. Antithrombin deficiency is divided into type I – a quantitative deficiency – and type II, a qualitative defect where the antithrombin protein produced is functionally abnormal. Type II deficiency is subclassified according to the site of the molecular defect, which may affect the reactive (thrombin-binding) site, heparin-binding site or both sites. This classification has clinical relevance, as the incidence of thrombosis is higher in association with type I and type II (reactive site) deficiency. Family studies show antithrombin deficiency to be a more severe disorder than protein C or protein S deficiency. The relative risk of VTE is around 25- to 50-fold for individuals with type I antithrombin deficiency. Low antithrombin levels are recorded in women using the combined oral contraceptive pill, patients on heparin treatment and those with acute thrombosis. Marked decreases in antithrombin levels are also observed in disseminated intravascular coagulation, liver disease and nephrotic syndrome.

### Prothrombin G20210A mutation

This genetic defect is due to a G→A transition at nucleotide 20210 in the 3∃-untranslated region of the prothrombin gene. This causes elevated plasma prothrombin levels and an increased risk of venous thrombosis. The prevalence of the mutation in Northern Europe is approximately 2% in the healthy population. The risk of venous thrombosis in carriers of the mutation is estimated to be around three times that of non-carriers.

### Dysfibrinogenaemia

This is a rare condition and most cases are asymptomatic and found by chance. In about 20% of cases there is an increased tendency to thromboembolism and in 25% there is a bleeding tendency.

### Elevated factor VIII

Factor VIII levels are determined by both genetic and environmental factors. Factor VIII levels above 150 IU/dl are associated with a sixfold increased risk of VTE compared with factor VIII levels of less than 100 IU/dl.

More recently, elevated levels of factors IX and XI have been associated with an increased risk of venous thrombosis.[2,3]

### Elevated homocysteine levels

Studies have demonstrated an approximately 2.5-fold increased risk of venous thrombosis in individuals with plasma homocysteine levels exceeding 18.5 μmol/l. Genetic analysis is not indicated as although the common thermolabile methylene tetrahydrofolate reductase variant contributes to hyperhomocysteinaemia, it is not itself associated with VTE. Other mutations are uncommon.

## The antiphospholipid syndrome

Antiphospholipid syndrome (APS) is a form of acquired, autoimmune thrombophilia. Patients have evidence of arterial/venous thrombotic events and/or pregnancy loss in association with antiphospholipid antibodies (APA). Diagnosis requires at least one of the clinical and one of the laboratory criteria shown in Table 6.2.

Studies suggest that around 30% of patients with systemic lupus erythematosis (SLE) develop APS. The detection of lupus anticoagulant in a patient with SLE predicts a 50% chance of a thrombotic event over 20 years follow-up. Measurements of APA are part of the routine investigations of women with recurrent pregnancy failure and APA are found in approximately 15% of cases.[4] Antiphospholipid antibodies (lupus anticoagulant and anticardiolipin antibodies) are found in 1%–5% of young, healthy control subjects. The

| Table 6.2 Sapporo classification criteria for the antiphospholipid syndrome | |
| --- | --- |
| **Clinical criteria** | |
| 1. Vascular thrombosis | Arterial, venous or small vessel thrombosis, in any organ or tissue |
| 2. Pregnancy morbidity | One or more unexplained death of normal fetus at or beyond the 10th week of gestation *or* |
| | One or more premature birth of normal neonate at or before the 34th week of gestation because of severe pre-eclampsia or eclampsia or severe placental insufficiency *or* |
| | Three or more unexplained consecutive spontaneous abortions before the 10th week of gestation |
| **Laboratory criteria** | |
| 1. Anticardiolipin antibody of immunoglobulin G (IgG) or IgM isotype in blood, present at medium or high titre, on two or more occasions, at least six weeks apart | |
| 2. Lupus anticoagulant present in the plasma on two or more occasions, at least six weeks apart | |

thrombotic risk associated with the incidental finding of APA appears to be low. Transient APA associated with infections such as syphilis are common and are not usually associated with thrombotic events. They may also be induced by drugs such as phenothiazines, which again are not generally associated with thrombosis.

## Investigation of thrombophilia

Indiscriminate thrombophilia screening of all individuals is unhelpful and not cost-effective; moreover, finding an abnormality often does not affect clinical management.[5] Investigation for inherited thrombophilia should be targeted at patients aged less than 50 years with an unusual site of thrombosis or recurrent venous thrombosis. Patients developing VTE in pregnancy or the post-partum period and those taking the combined oral contraceptive pill also warrant investigation as the detection of defects is high in this group. The chances of finding an inherited thrombophilic defect are much lower if the patient is older or the thrombotic event is provoked. A scheme for investigating patients for thrombophilia is illustrated in Figure 6.2.

Venous thromboembolism is common and associated with a significant risk of recurrence and its treatment is associated with significant bleeding complications. On standard anticoagulant therapy, major haemorrhage occurs at a rate of around 1% per year of treatment and one-quarter of these bleeds are fatal.[6] The ability to identify patients at high and low risk of thrombosis would help to optimize therapeutic decisions. Identification of an inherited thrombophilic defect can be helpful in decision making for that individual and family members. The risk of thrombosis related to the contraceptive pill has now been shown to be significantly increased in affected family members of families with thrombophilia. Similarly, the risk of thrombosis in association with surgery, trauma or immobility is significantly elevated, and prophylaxis for these situations is recommended.

Investigation for thrombophilia in most cases of venous thrombosis is unlikely to lead to altered clinical management. Recurrence of VTE after stopping oral anticoagulant treatment has not been shown to be predictable by thrombophilia testing, hence duration of anticoagulation should generally be the same for patients with and without labo-

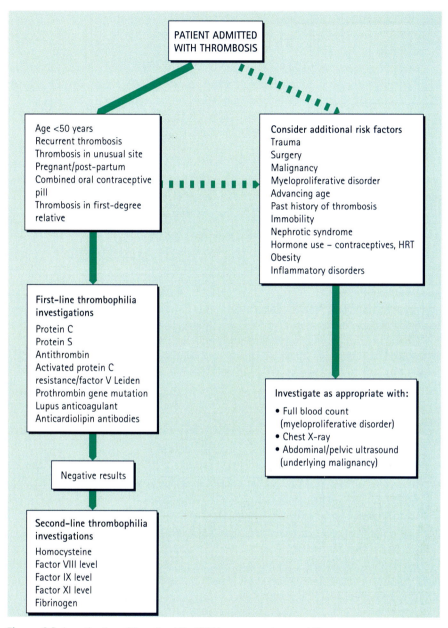

**Figure 6.2** Investigation of thrombophilia. HRT, hormone replacement therapy.

ratory evidence of thrombophilia. There is also no evidence that the detection of an inherited thrombophilic defect alters the choice or intensity of anticoagulant.[7]

Patients with high-risk thrombophilic defects (e.g. type I or type II reactive-site antithrombin deficiency or combined defects) should be assessed individually by a haematologist regarding extension of the usual period of anticoagulation as data are conflicting.

The timing of laboratory tests for heritable thrombophilia (for example, assays of antithrombin, protein C and protein S) is important as the levels are influenced by several factors. In particular they are affected by the acute thrombotic state, anticoagulant use, pregnancy and hormone therapy. Also, finding a thrombophilic abnormality hardly ever influences the management of an acute thrombotic event. Testing is therefore best performed at least 4 weeks after completion of a course of anticoagulation. However, if deemed necessary before this point, then it is essential that the individual interpreting the screen is aware of the presence and potential influence of acquired factors on the test results. Molecular tests for factor V Leiden and the prothrombin 20210A allele are unaffected by such factors. It is strongly recommended that thrombophilia testing is supervised by and results are interpreted by an experienced clinician who is aware of all relevant factors that may influence test results in each individual.

# Recent Developments

### New inherited thrombophilic risk factors

Protein Z-dependent protease inhibitor (ZPI) is a serpin that inhibits the activated coagulation factors X and XI. As for antithrombin, deficiency of ZPI could have relevant thrombotic consequences. Results of studies analysing mutations in the ZPI gene suggest an association between ZPI deficiency and venous thrombosis, with carriers of a particular polymorphism having a threefold risk of thrombosis and a familial history of thrombosis.[8]

Recently, the frequency of a polymorphism of factor VII-activating protease (Marburg I polymorphism) was shown to be significantly increased in patients with VTE and the variant acted as an independent risk factor, although it has been shown to be only a mild risk factor for recurrent VTE.[9]

### Thrombophilia and pregnancy complications

It is widely accepted that women with a history of recurrent miscarriage/stillbirth should be screened for APA. In APS, placental thrombosis and infarction occurs with related fetal loss. Current evidence suggests a similar pathogenesis in inherited thrombophilia and the presence of a thrombophilic defect does increase the risk of fetal loss and other pregnancy complications such as pre-eclampsia or intrauterine growth retardation. However, the role of testing for heritable defects is not clear-cut as there is uncertainty as to whether this should alter management, for example by giving thromboprophylaxis.

A recent study treated pregnant women known to have inherited thrombophilia with thromboprophylaxis using low-molecular-weight heparin. Fetal loss rates were significantly reduced in deficient women receiving thromboprophylaxis compared to those without prophylaxis.[10] The data suggest that anticoagulant treatment during pregnancy reduces the high fetal loss rate in women with hereditary deficiencies of antithrombin, protein C or protein S.

# Conclusion

Thrombophilia screening is only of value in selected cases and should not be carried out routinely as many patients who carry an inherited thrombophilic defect never have a thrombosis. Testing should be targeted at patients with specific risk factors but even then clinical management rarely changes.

# Further Reading

1 Walker ID, Greaves M, Preston FE. Investigation and management of heritable thrombophilia. *Br J Haematol* 2001; **114**: 512–28.

2 Meijers JC, Tekelenburg WL, Bouma BN, Bertina RM, Rosendaal FR. High levels of coagulation factor XI as a risk factor for venous thrombosis. *N Engl J Med* 2000; **342**: 696–701.

3 Weltermann A, Eichinger S, Bialonczyk C, *et al.* The risk of recurrent venous thromboembolism among patients with high factor IX levels. *J Thromb Haemost* 2003; **1**: 28–32.

4 Robertson B, Greaves M. Antiphospholipid syndrome: an evolving story. *Blood Rev* 2006; **20**: 201–12.

5 Baglin TJ. Thrombophilia testing: what do we think the tests mean and what should we do with the results? *Clin Pathol* 2000; **53**: 167–70.

6 Palareti G, Leali N, Coccheri S, *et al.* Bleeding complications of oral anticoagulant treatment: an inception-cohort, prospective collaborative study (ISCOAT). *Lancet* 1996; **348**: 423–8.

7 Christiansen SC, Cannegieter SC, Koster T, Vandenbroucke JP, Rosendaal FR. Thrombophilia, clinical factors, and recurrent venous thrombotic events. *JAMA* 2005; **293**: 2352–61.

8 Razzari C, Martinelli I, Bucciarelli P, Viscardi Y, Biguzzi E. Polymorphisms of the protein Z-dependent protease inhibitor (ZPI) gene and the risk of venous thromboembolism. *Thromb Haemost* 2006; **95**: 909–10.

9 Gulesserian T, Hiron G, Endler G, Eichinger S, Wagner O, Kyrle PA. Marburg I polymorphism of factor VII-activating protease and risk of recurrent venous thromboembolism. *Thromb Haemost* 2006; **95**: 65–7.

10 Folkeringa N, Brouwer JL, Korteweg FJ, *et al.* Reduction of high fetal loss rate by anticoagulant treatment during pregnancy in antithrombin, protein C or protein S deficient women. *Br J Haematol* 2007; **136**: 656–61.

# Red Cell Disorders and Aplastic Anaemia

**PROBLEM**

## 07 The investigation of anaemia and the anaemia of chronic disease

## Case History

A 55-year-old woman with rheumatoid arthritis is referred to the haematology outpatient department by her General Practitioner. She consulted him because of symptoms of profound fatigue and tinnitus and a routine full blood count had revealed her to be anaemic. Haemoglobin was 10.3 g/dl, mean cell volume (MCV) 82 fl, white cell count 5.6 (neutrophils 3.5, lymphocytes 2.1) $\times 10^9$/l and platelets 287 $\times 10^9$/l. Her doctor could not establish a clear-cut cause for this lady's anaemia and has sought further advice.

**What is the clinical approach to managing this patient?**

**What investigations should be performed?**

## Background

As in any other clinical scenario, the investigation of this patient hinges on an accurate history and examination. In terms of causes of anaemia, the most common by far is iron deficiency and the likelihood of this as an explanation should be fairly clear by paying close attention to diet history, enquiring for gastrointestinal symptoms and obtaining a gynaecological history in females. A lot of information can be gleaned from the full blood count result, the key parameter being red blood cell (RBC) size. In terms of aetiology, the classification of anaemias (Figure 7.1) is best approached based around the MCV. Clearly in uncomplicated iron deficiency, patients will have a microcytic hypochromic blood film, and it is debatable whether such patients need referral to a specialist haematology clinic. The common causes of iron deficiency are related to occult gastrointestinal blood loss or menorrhagia and the appropriate management of such cases lies with the appropriate specialty.

However, this case presents one of the commonest diagnostic dilemmas – the patient with a normocytic anaemia in whom haematinic levels are normal and there is no morphological evidence of bone marrow failure or haemolysis. It is a common problem, the presence of which increases with age. Often patients are asymptomatic, the condition being discovered by 'routine' laboratory tests. Although all causes of microcytic and macrocytic anaemias can on occasion present with a normocytic anaemia, often in this situation one is dealing with a decreased production of normal-sized RBCs, as occurs in the anaemia of chronic disease (ACD) but also in aplastic anaemia. A similar appearance can occur in an uncompensated increase in plasma volume, for example in pregnancy or fluid overload. Anaemia of chronic disease is thought to be the most common form of normocytic anaemia and probably the second most common form of anaemia worldwide after iron-deficiency anaemia. It is often a disease of exclusion and the pathogenesis is usually multifactorial and thought to be related to hypoactivity of the bone marrow with relative inadequate production of erythropoietin (EPO) or a poor response to EPO. There is probably also reduced RBC survival. The clinical history and examination will often identify the underlying chronic disorder, which includes a wide range of inflammatory conditions including arthritis, infections and malignant disease. Iron studies usually reveal a decreased serum iron level but with a decreased transferrin level (rather than a raised level as seen in iron deficiency) and a normal or elevated serum ferritin.

# Recent Developments

### Understanding the pathophysiology of ACD

In ACD there is an impaired erythropoietic response related to impaired mobilization and utilization of reticuloendothelial iron. This is associated with a blunted EPO response and a relative resistance to EPO. There is also reduced RBC survival, which may be due to selective haemolyisis of young RBCs due to EPO deficiency. The causes of ACD may be related to altered inflammatory regulation by sex hormones and reduced catabolism of inflammatory cytokines. As a result, protracted elevation of interleukin-6 (IL-6) and tumour necrosis factor α (TNF-α) can be seen in the plasma of elderly patients after exposure to inflammatory stimuli and this may be a common mechanism for the production of anaemia in chronic illness, particularly in elderly subjects.[1]

Recently, the iron regulatory hormone hepcidin has been proposed as the mediator of the iron abnormalities seen in ACD.[2,3] Hepcidin is an acute phase peptide whose production causes degradation of the iron export protein ferroportin. Iron is retained in reticuloendothelial cells and is therefore unavailable for erythropoiesis. Murine experiments

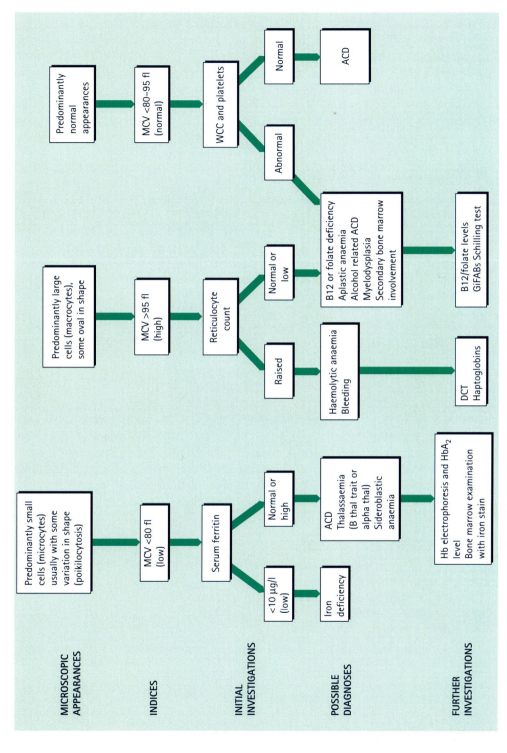

**Figure 7.1** The approach to the anaemic patient. DCT, direct Coombs' test; GiFAbs, growth inhibitory factor antibodies; Hb, haemoglobin; thal, thalassaemia; WCC, white cell count.

have shown that, even in the absence of inflammation, transgenic mice that have repressed hepcidin suffer from severe iron-refractory anaemia. Additionally, it has been shown that patients with large hepatic adenomas may autonomously produce this peptide and also develop severe iron-refractory anaemia, which is reversed by the resection of the adenoma. It is likely that chronic hepcidin production in the setting of an inflammatory stimulus will induce anaemia by inducing a sequestration of iron and hypoferremia. This overproduction occurs via inflammatory cytokines, especially IL-6. Greater understanding of the role of hepcidin in the development of ACD may, through specific drug development to block its action, lead to pharmacological therapy for ACD in the future.

### Treatment

Treatment of this condition is troublesome. The adage usually is that attention be given to the underlying disorder. In the very specific area of ACD associated with renal disease, which is more appropriately classified as a separate cause of a normocytic anaemia, there is a relative underproduction of EPO and EPO therapy can transform the quality of life of these individuals. However, there are several reports in the literature of the effectiveness of EPO in ACD not associated with renal disease, with some reports suggesting that routine iron supplementation may enhance the response.[4]

## Conclusion

The possible causes of anaemia in a middle-aged lady are many but iron deficiency remains the most important one to exclude and appropriately investigate (particularly for occult gastrointestinal neoplasm) if this is suspected, despite the presence of any coincidental inflammatory disorder. Anaemia of chronic disease is often a diagnosis of exclusion, but it is a very frequent clinical problem with no clear-cut way forward in terms of management other than addressing the underlying clinical problem. However, the likelihood of pharmacological intervention in the future (other than with EPO therapy) may be greater with the developing understanding of the mechanisms involved.

## Further Reading

1  Ershler WB, Keller ET. Age-associated increased interleukin-6 gene expression, late-life diseases, and frailty. *Annu Rev Med* 2000; **51**: 245–70.

2  Ganz T. Hepcidin, a key regulator of iron metabolism and mediator of anemia of inflammation. *Blood* 2003; **102**: 783–8.

3  Dallalio G, Law E, Means Jr RT. Hepcidin inhibits in vitro erythroid colony formation at reduced erythropoietin concentrations. *Blood* 2006; **107**: 2702–4.

4  Arndt U, Kaltwasser JP, Gottschalk R, Hoelzer D, Möller B. Correction of iron-deficient erythropoiesis in the treatment of anemia of chronic disease with recombitant human erythropoietin. *Ann Hematol* 2005; **84**: 159–66.

**PROBLEM**

# 08 Aplastic anaemia

## Case History

A 32-year-old man presented with a two-month history of increasing tiredness and shortness of breath. His exercise tolerance reduced over the two-month period from regularly running eight kilometres to only being able to walk. Over the last week he had recurrent nose bleeds and spontaneous bruising. At the time of his presentation he had had no raised temperatures. Two months prior to his presentation he had a diarrhoeal illness after travelling to India and received treatment with metronidazole for presumed giardiasis. There was no other relevant previous or family history. His three sisters and brother were all alive and well. He was on no drugs. On examination he had some bruising, a petechial rash and two small fundal haemorrhages. There was no lymphadenopathy or hepatosplenomegaly. At presentation his white cell count was $1.3 \times 10^9/l$, neutrophils 0.6 $\times 10^9/l$, haemoglobin 5.1 g/dl and platelets $6 \times 10^9/l$. A blood film was consistent with pancytopenia and had no diagnostic features.

**What are the most likely causes of his pancytopenia?**

**What investigations would you perform?**

**What treatment would you give over the next 24 hours?**

## Background

The differential diagnosis includes bone marrow replacement by leukaemia (acute myeloid leukaemia or acute lymphoblastic leukaemia – the lack of blasts in the blood film is unusual but is observed in rare cases, for example in acute promyelocytic leukaemia) or aplastic anaemia (usually idiopathic or secondary to drugs, hepatitis, etc.).[1] Aplastic anaemia is most likely in view of the prior history of illness treated with antibiotics (although metronidazole is not a very well-recognized cause of aplastic anaemia, this side-effect has been reported), the lack of abnormalities on the blood film and the profound anaemia with relatively few signs (suggesting a slow onset). Other unlikely causes would be pernicious anaemia (unlikely due to the patient's age and gender), myelodysplastic syndrome (more common in the elderly and a morphologically abnormal blood film would be expected) and metastatic carcinoma (expectation of a leuco-erythroblastic blood film).

The diagnosis of aplastic anaemia was established with a bone marrow aspirate and trephine biopsy (Figure 8.1). There was no increase in blasts in the marrow and cytogenetic analysis revealed a normal male karyotype (46, XY). Flow cytometry revealed the normal expression of glycosyl phosphatidyl inositol-linked antigens, excluding a diagnosis of paroxysmal nocturnal haemoglobinuria (PNH).[2] He has severe aplastic anaemia according to the Camitta criteria.[3] His initial management included the transfusion of platelets to maintain a level over $50 \times 10^9/l$ in view of his fundal haemorrhages (a finding that indicates a potential risk of intracranial haemorrhage and necessitates intensive correction of the haemostatic defect – in this case thrombocytopenia). He was transfused with six units of packed red blood cells. The patient and all his siblings were tissue typed – the brother was human leukocyte antigen (HLA)-identical with the patient.

**What are the treatment options?**

**What is his prognosis?**

The treatment options lie between an allogeneic stem cell transplant[4] from his HLA-identical sibling or immune suppressive therapy with antilymphocyte globulin and ciclosporin.[5] The outcome for transplantation in severe aplastic anaemia is dependent on the age of the patient (older patients having a higher mortality and an increased risk of acute and chronic graft-versus-host disease [GvHD]) and the type of marrow donor

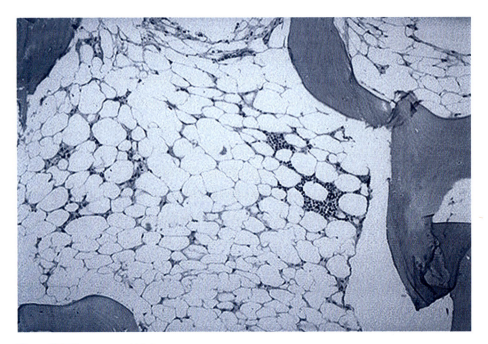

**Figure 8.1** Bone marrow histology.

(HLA-identical sibling transplants have a better outcome than matched unrelated donor transplants). For patients between 30 and 40 years of age the 5-year survival following a transplant from an HLA-identical donor is in the region of 65%, with approximately 30% of patients suffering from chronic GvHD.[6] A distinct advantage for transplantation over immune suppressive therapy is that the disease is cured with no risk of late haematological clonal disorders such as myelodysplastic syndrome or PNH.[7]

Immune suppressive therapy using the combination of antilymphocyte globulin (ALG, or antithymocyte globulin [ATG]) with ciclosporin is associated with response rates of approximately 80% with a 5-year survival of approximately 75%.[8] After immune suppressive therapy, patients usually need to receive continued blood-product support until attaining a response to treatment, which usually occurs between 4 and 6 months from therapy. In most patients, a second cycle of ALG and ciclosporin is required 6 months after the first. Ciclosporin is usually weaned about 6 months after a response but a minority of patients require continued low doses of ciclosporin. Relapse may occur after immune suppressive therapy in approximately 10% of cases. Whilst the early mortality of immune suppressive therapy is much lower than with allogeneic transplantation, the major problems are a proportion of patients who do not respond (approximately 20% of patients) and the risk of late clonal disease, such as myelodysplastic syndrome (10%), clinically significant PNH (15%) and, occasionally, acute myeloid leukaemia (<5%).

# Recent Developments

1 Importance of the telomere and telomerase in the pathophysiology of inherited aplastic anaemia.

2 Improvements in outcome following allogeneic bone marrow transplantation (BMT) have meant that BMT from an HLA-identical sibling is the preferred treatment for severe aplastic anaemia up to 40 years.

3 Haematopoietc growth factors (G-CSF or erythropoietin) are not routinely recommended in the immune suppressive treatment of aplastic anaemia.

4 Horse ALG (Lymphoglobuline, Genzyme) has now been withdrawn and replaced by rabbit ATG (Thymoglobuline, Genzyme) which should be used for the initial course of immunosuppressive therapy.

# Conclusion

After discussion with the patient and his family it was decided to treat him with immune suppressive therapy. He received his first course of ALG (horse derived), which he tolerated very well, 4 weeks after his presentation. He received oral prednisolone, to prevent serum sickness, which was reduced and stopped in the first 4 weeks after ALG. He started ciclosporin immediately after completing his ALG. He had a minimal response in that he became platelet-transfusion independent after 4 months but continued to receive red cell transfusions. After 6 months he received a second course of ALG (rabbit derived) and continued ciclosporin. After a further 6 months he remained red cell-transfusion dependent and therefore had danazol added to the ciclosporin. He became transfusion

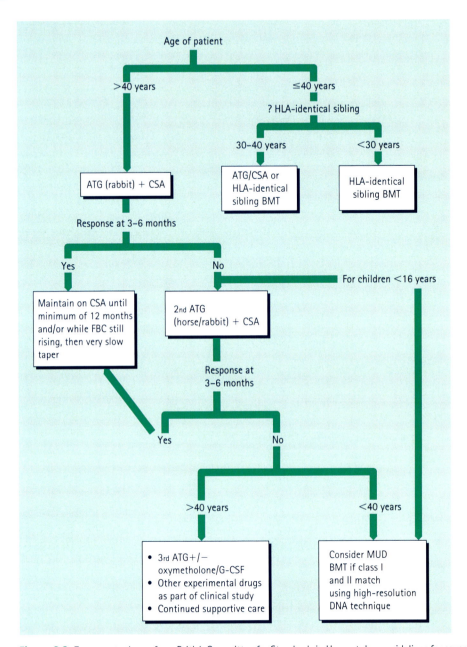

**Figure 8.2** Treatment schema from British Committee for Standards in Haematology guidelines for severe acquired aplastic anaemia.[9] BMT, bone marrow transplantation; CSA, ciclosporin; FBC, full blood count; G-CSF, granulocyte colony stimulating factor; MUD, matched unrelated donor.

independent 3 months later. His blood count became normal 2 years after his initial presentation. In the 18 months immediately after his diagnosis he received in the region of 130 units of packed cells and his serum ferritin was over 5000 ng/ml. Iron chelation with desferrioxamine had been avoided due to his thrombocytopenia. However, after his recovery he underwent venesections every 2 weeks to remove his excess iron. His vene-sections continued for 3 years until his serum ferritin level was normal. He stopped dana-zol after 2 years and stopped ciclosporin after 4 years. No late clonal haematopoietic disorders, such as PNH and myelodysplastic syndrome, have occurred.

Historically, the diagnosis of severe aplastic anaemia had a grave prognosis. However, the advent of both allogeneic stem cell transplantation and immune suppressive therapy (Figure 8.2) has improved survival to the region of 80%. For patients under 30 years of age and with an HLA-identical sibling, transplant is generally performed; for those over 40 years of age, immune suppressive therapy is preferred. The decision of whether to transplant or not is most difficult for those between the ages of 30 and 40 years.

# Further Reading

1   Young NS, Calado RT, Scheinberg P. Current concepts in the pathophysiology and treatment of aplastic anemia. *Blood* 2006; **108**: 2509–19.

2   Hill A, Richards SJ, Hillmen P. Recent developments in the understanding and management of paroxysmal nocturnal haemoglobinuria. *Br J Haematol* 2007; **137**: 181–92.

3   Camitta BM, Thomas ED, Nathan DG, *et al.* Severe aplastic anaemia; a prospective study of the effect of early marrow transplantation on acute mortality. *Blood* 1976; **48**: 63–70.

4   Bacigalupo A, Brand R, Oneto R, *et al.* Treatment of acquired severe aplastic anaemia: bone marrow transplantation compared with immunosuppressive therapy – The European Group for Blood and Marrow Transplantation experience. *Semin Hematol* 2000; **37**: 69–80.

5   Frickhofen N, Heimpel H, Kaltwasser JP, Schrezenmeier H. Antithymocyte globulin with or without cyclosporin A: 11-year follow-up of a randomized trial comparing treatments of aplastic anaemia. *Blood* 2003; **101**: 1236–42.

6   Passweg JR, Socié G, Hinterberger W, *et al.* Bone marrow transplantation for severe aplastic anaemia: has outcome improved? *Blood* 1997; **90**: 858–64.

7   Socié G, Rosenfeld S, Frickhofen N, Gluckman E, Tichelli A. Late clonal diseases of treated aplastic anaemia. *Semin Hematol* 2000; **37**: 91–101.

8   Marsh J, Schrezenmeier H, Marin P, *et al.* Prospective randomized multicenter study comparing cyclosporin alone versus the combination of antithymocyte globulin and cyclosporin for treatment of patients with nonsevere aplastic anemia: a report from the European Blood and Marrow Transplant (EBMT) Severe Aplastic Anaemia Working Party. *Blood* 1999; **93**: 2191–5.

9   Marsh JC, Ball SE, Cavenagh J, *et al.* Guidelines for the diagnosis and management of acquired aplastic anaemia. *Br J Haematol* 2009; **147**: 43–70.

# 09 Paroxysmal nocturnal haemoglobinuria

## Case History

A 31-year-old woman, who had previously been well, presented to her General Practitioner after 'passing blood in her urine'. It was assumed that she had passed a renal stone and had now recovered. She had a similar episode 5 months later where she passed blood for 2 days. She was then referred to a urologist who performed a variety of investigations but found no abnormality to explain her haematuria. She had no further problems until she presented again 12 months later with a prolonged episode of haematuria, symptoms of anaemia, abdominal pain and difficulty in swallowing. At this time her full blood count was abnormal: white blood cells $5.4 \times 10^9$/l; neutrophils $2.2 \times 10^9$/l; haemoglobin 6.8 g/dl; mean cell volume 69 fl; platelets $123 \times 10^9$/l.

**What diagnosis would explain all of her features?**

**What tests would you perform to establish the diagnosis?**

**What other tests would you perform?**

**What is the most feared complication of this disorder?**

## Background

The diagnosis that explains all of the symptoms and abnormalities is paroxysmal nocturnal haemoglobinuria (PNH).[1] The red urine is actually haemoglobinuria not haematuria (there are no intact red cells in the urine – a simple test is to allow the urine to stand for approximately 30 minutes and haematuria will settle whereas haemoglobinuria will not). Patients with PNH have chronic intravascular haemolysis due to the uncontrolled effect of complement on the abnormal red blood cells and this results in intermittent episodes of haemoglobinuria (particularly in the mornings), anaemia due to haemolysis and to iron loss in the urine, and symptoms associated with free haemoglobin in the plasma (dysphagia, abdominal pain and severe lethargy out of keeping with the degree of anaemia).

The diagnostic test for PNH is flow cytometry to assess the expression of glycosyl phosphatidyl inositol (GPI)-linked antigens on the surface of the blood cells (Figure 9.1).[2] Flow cytometry was performed using samples from our patient and this confirmed the diagnosis of PNH: 99.5% of her neutrophils were GPI deficient (CD59–, CD16$^{low}$ = PNH phenotype) and 37% of her red cells were GPI deficient (CD59– and CD55–).

The other tests that should be performed are on markers of haemolysis (reticulocyte count, lactate dehydrogenase, haptoglobins) and haematinics (including folic acid and

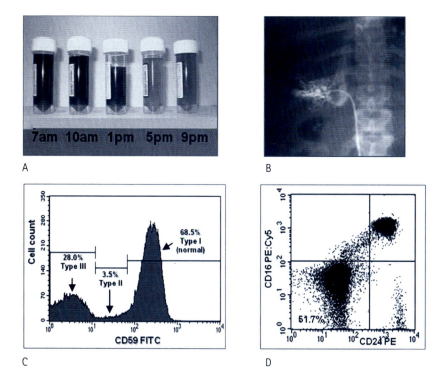

**Figure 9.1** (A) Urine passed through the day, showing initially intense haemoglobinuria which clears through the day. (B) Hepatic vein thrombosis. (C) Red cell flow cytometry demonstrating deficiency of CD59 (a GPI-linked antigen) diagnostic of PNH. This case has 28.0% red cells with complete deficiency of CD59 and 3.5% with a partial deficiency. (D) Neutrophil flow cytometry demonstrating 51.7% neutrophils with deficiency of two GPI-linked antigens (CD16 and CD24).

ferritin). The patient may also require an abdominal ultrasound scan to exclude occult thrombosis causing her abdominal pain and an upper gastrointestinal endoscopy in view of her abdominal pain and iron deficiency.

The most feared complication of PNH is venous thrombosis, particularly affecting the intra-abdominal veins or the cerebral veins. Patients with large PNH clones (over 50% PNH neutrophils) are at greatest risk, with approximately one-half of patients experiencing venous thrombosis at some stage.[3–5] There is evidence that primary prophylaxis with warfarin significantly reduces the thrombotic risk, although it is clear that warfarin is not totally protective and is ineffective after the occurrence of the first thrombosis (that is, as secondary prophylaxis).[3]

The patient received a two-unit blood transfusion (these were not washed red cells, as was the practice in PNH in the past, as this has been shown to be unnecessary as long as blood of the same blood group is used). A Doppler ultrasound scan of her abdomen revealed no evidence of thrombosis. She was iron deficient but oral iron replacement had no impact on her haemoglobin level. She commenced folic acid, as is routine for patients with haemolytic anaemia. After counselling she commenced prophylaxis with warfarin aiming for an International Normalized Ratio (INR) of between 2.0 and 3.0. She continued to require transfusions every 6 to 8 weeks. The patient did not tolerate warfarin (she did not like the regular monitoring) and, after discussion, was changed from warfarin to aspirin (there is no good evidence that aspirin prevents thrombosis in PNH). Unfortunately, 9 months after stopping her warfarin she developed skin lesions over her chest and these were shown to be due to dermal vein thrombosis. She was heparinized and recommenced on warfarin. The following month she was readmitted with abdominal pain and vomiting which was shown to be due to duodenal oedema secondary to mesenteric vein thrombosis. During that admission, a left subclavian vein thrombosis was diagnosed. She was eventually discharged but was readmitted a month later with further abdominal pain and swelling.

**What is the likely cause of her abdominal pain and swelling?**

**What tests would you perform to establish the diagnosis?**

**How would you manage this problem?**

**Are there any specific treatments for PNH that may have an impact on the haemolysis and thrombosis seen in PNH?**

The most likely cause of her symptoms is the development of hepatic vein thrombosis or a Budd–Chiari syndrome with abdominal pain and ascites. This was confirmed by abdominal ultrasound and with a hepatic venogram. She was initially thrombolysed with tissue plasminogen activator infused both locally to the thrombus and systemically.[6] This resulted in a significant improvement but, unfortunately, 3 weeks later she had a recurrence. Her ascites was then relieved by a transjugular intrahepatic portosystemic shunt (TIPSS).

The patient's condition stabilized after an episode of both renal and hepatic dysfunction, although she had several admissions with recurrent abdominal painful crises and continued to require two to three units of red cells every week. During this period she also had a left internal jugular vein thrombosis and multiple pulmonary emboli. Therefore she had suffered six different thrombotic events over a 4-month period despite receiving warfarin with a 'therapeutic' INR.

The patient then became eligible for a clinical trial of the anti-complement monoclonal antibody, eculizumab. She was initially treated with weekly 600 mg infusions of eculizumab for 4 weeks and thereafter with 900 mg every 2 weeks. She has now been on eculizumab for over 4 years with no further thromboses, requires transfusions infrequently (approximately every 3 months) and has had no further symptoms of her PNH or admissions to hospital. She remains on eculizumab and is now working full-time with relatively little inconvenience to her daily life.

# Recent Developments

### Flow cytometry

Flow cytometry has superseded the Ham–Dacie test as the diagnostic test for PNH. The Ham–Dacie test, which was first described in the 1930s, depends on the excessive sensitivity to complement of PNH red cells. However, the Ham–Dacie test is only, at best, semiquantitative and can result in false-positive and false-negative results. In contrast, flow cytometry is less likely to give the incorrect result and is also quantitative for the size of the PNH cell populations in all haematopoietic lineages.

## Treatment of PNH

Until 2007, PNH was treated with supportive measures as there was no effective therapy to control the haemolysis nor any effective therapy for established thrombotic complications. Bone marrow transplantation is a curative approach but has a very high transplant-related mortality in published series and only a minority of patients have suitable matched donors.[7] The anti-complement antibody, eculizumab, was approved for the treatment of PNH in 2007 on the basis of a randomized, placebo-controlled trial and two small phase II studies. These trials demonstrated that eculizumab results in a marked reduction in intravascular haemolysis, with many patients becoming transfusion independent and attaining very significant improvements in quality of life and symptoms.[8–10] In addition, recent evidence indicates that eculizumab has a profound influence on the thrombotic risk in PNH and therefore might be anticipated to improve survival.[11]

# Conclusion

Our patient has several typical features of PNH. First of all, many patients are investigated for 'haematuria', often several times before it is realized that they actually have haemoglobinuria. Her initial thrombosis is in a classical site and the series of apparently unrelated life-threatening thromboses is again typical and frequently heralds a fulminant course. Her response to eculizumab has been impressive, with the likelihood that eculizumab has broken the cycle of thrombosis that she had entered despite 'adequate' anticoagulation.

# Further Reading

1 Hill A, Richards SJ, Hillmen P. Recent developments in the understanding and management of paroxysmal nocturnal haemoglobinuria. *Br J Haematol* 2007; **137**: 181–92.

2 Richards SJ, Rawstron AC, Hillmen P. The application of flow cytometry to the diagnosis of paroxysmal nocturnal hemoglobinuria. *Cytometry* 2000; **42**: 223–33.

3 Hall C, Richards S, Hillmen P. Primary prophylaxis with warfarin prevents thrombosis in paroxysmal nocturnal hemoglobinuria (PNH). *Blood* 2003; **102**: 3587–91.

4 Moyo VM, Mukhina GL, Garrett ES, Brodsky RA. Natural history of paroxysmal nocturnal haemoglobinuria using modern diagnostic assays. *Br J Haematol* 2004; **126**: 133–8.

5 Nishimura J, Kanakura Y, Ware RE, *et al.* Clinical course and flow cytometric analysis of paroxysmal nocturnal hemoglobinuria in the United States and Japan. *Medicine (Baltimore)* 2004; **83**: 193–207.

6 McMullin MF, Hillmen P, Jackson J, Ganly P, Luzzatto L. Tissue plasminogen activator for hepatic vein thrombosis in paroxysmal nocturnal haemoglobinuria. *J Intern Med* 1994; **235**: 85–9.

7 Saso R, Marsh J, Cevreska L, *et al.* Bone marrow transplants for paroxysmal nocturnal haemoglobinuria. *Br J Haematol* 1999; **104**: 392–6.

8 Hillmen P, Hall C, Marsh JC, *et al.* Effect of eculizumab on hemolysis and transfusion requirements in patients with paroxysmal nocturnal hemoglobinuria. *N Engl J Med* 2004; **350**: 552–9.

9 Hillmen P, Young NS, Schubert J, *et al.* The complement inhibitor eculizumab in paroxysmal nocturnal hemoglobinuria. *N Engl J Med* 2006; **355**: 1233–43.

10 Hill A, Hillmen P, Richards SJ, *et al.* Sustained response and long-term safety of eculizumab in paroxysmal nocturnal hemoglobinuria. *Blood* 2005; **106**: 2559–65.

11 Hillmen P, Muus P, Dührsen U, *et al.* Effect of the complement inhibitor eculizumab on thromboembolism in patients with paroxysmal nocturnal hemoglobinuria. *Blood* 2007; **110**: 4123–8.

## PROBLEM

# 10 Sickle cell disease

## Case History

A 24-year-old student from Ghana attends Accident and Emergency with severe chest wall pains. He gives a history of sickle cell disease (SCD) and has been admitted to another hospital with crises at least twice in the past year. He thinks the pain is due to another crisis and his usual analgesics do not alleviate it. His haemoglobin is 8.5 g/dl, mean cell volume 94 fl, white blood cells (WBC) $12.3 \times 10^9/l$, platelets $450 \times 10^9/l$ and reticulocyte count is $325 \times 10^9/l$. The blood film shows prominent sickle cells, target cells, basophilic stippling and Howell–Jolly bodies and a sickle solubility test is positive. His oxygen saturation is 98% on air. A chest X-ray (CXR) is normal.

**What is your initial management plan?**

## Background

The sickling syndromes are genetic conditions in which at least one β-globin gene allele on chromosome 11 carries the $\beta^S$ (Val6Glu) mutation. A single nucleotide change in the β-globin gene leads to substitution of valine for glutamic acid at position 6 of the β-globin chain. Conformational change upon deoxygenation of the resultant haemoglobin (haemoglobin S; HbS) exposes a hydrophobic area at the site of the $\beta^6$ valine. Interaction with a complementary site on a β subunit of another haemoglobin tetramer ($\alpha_2\beta^S_2$) initiates polymerization, which causes deformation, or sickling, of the red blood cell (RBC).

The homozygous state, HbSS or sickle cell anaemia, is one of the most severe forms of SCD and is the most common (around 70% in the UK);[1] HbSC compound heterozygotes account for the majority of the remainder. Other compound heterozygous states can also produce SCD (HbS/β⁰ thalassaemia, HbS/β⁺ thalassaemia [including HbS/Hb Lepore], HbS/D$^{Punjab}$ and HbS/O$^{Arab}$).

The heterozygous state (HbAS) is not associated with sickling at normal oxygenation.

## Prevalence

DNA studies have led to the belief that the sickle cell mutation has arisen independently in several different populations. Falciparum malaria then acted as a selection factor, as sickle cell trait, not SCD, confers a survival advantage against malaria. This selection pressure has resulted in high frequencies of the mutant gene in areas of high malarial transmission, e.g. sub-Saharan Africa, India, Saudi Arabia and Mediterranean countries. In west African countries, such as Ghana and Nigeria, the frequency of the trait is 15% to 30%.[2] Subsequent migration has raised the frequency of the gene in other parts of the world.

## Pathophysiology

The primary event is polymerization of HbS within the red cell. The resultant sickling leads to vaso-occlusion and it is this manifestation that differentiates SCD from other haemolytic anaemias.

The tendency to polymerization of haemoglobin within the red cell depends on a number of factors including:

- oxygen saturation;
- percentage of HbS within the cell;
- percentage of fetal haemoglobin (HbF) within the cell;
- cell hydration.

Cycles of oxygenation and deoxygenation of RBCs produce repeated sickling and unsickling, leading to RBC membrane damage. This leads to red cell dehydration, increased rate of red cell breakdown (haemolytic anaemia) and the formation of a very short-lived, but continuously formed, subpopulation of very high density, irreversibly sickled RBCs.

## Clinical features

The phenotype of SCD varies from one of very few problems to a shortened life of ill health punctuated by frequent, painful and often life-threatening crises. The clinical features reflect the pathophysiology, with vaso-occlusive crises being the hallmark of SCD. These usually manifest themselves as severe pains in the bones, joints or abdomen. Triggers for crises include infection, dehydration, stress and cold, but often no cause is found. Children may get dactylitis: painful, swollen hands and feet. Newborns have a higher level of HbF and clinical manifestations are usually not apparent in the first few months of life.

In addition to the uncomplicated vaso-occlusive crisis there may be severe crises which include:

- acute chest syndrome;
- aplastic crisis – due to parvovirus B19 infection;
- haemolytic crisis – may be drug induced, secondary to infection or associated with glucose 6-phosphate dehydrogenase deficiency;
- priapism;
- sequestration crisis (usually children) – pooling of large volumes of blood in the spleen and/or liver;
- stroke.

## Laboratory features

The diagnosis is confirmed by haemoglobin electrophoresis, high-performance liquid chromatography and isoelectric focusing, which can detect the presence of abnormal haemoglobins. Evidence of haemolytic anaemia – low haemoglobin, reticulocytosis, elevated lactate dehydrogenase and bilirubin, and low haptoglobin – is present in the major forms of SCD.

This patient's haemoglobin is low, there is evidence of haemolytic anaemia and there are sickle cells on the blood film. Therefore he has SCD and appears to be having an acute painful crisis. He is rapidly assessed and hospital admission is arranged to ensure adequate analgesia and monitoring for life-threatening complications. Two days after admission he becomes unwell with a pyrexia of 39°C. He is tachypnoeic and his oxygen saturation is 92%. A repeat CXR shows new pulmonary infiltrates.

**What is the likely diagnosis and how should it be managed?**

## Pain management

In 1999 the American Pain Society published an evidence-based guideline for the management of acute and chronic pain in SCD.[3] However, there are no large controlled trails of analgesic regimens in SCD and smaller trials have failed to demonstrate an optimal regimen.

A number of guidelines recommend that severe pain should be treated promptly, after rapid clinical assessment (see algorithm in Figure 10.1). Attention should be paid to prior analgesic history and response to treatment should be closely monitored. The aim is to achieve rapid pain control. Once pain is controlled, the underlying cause can be assessed. If pain is thought to be not typical of a crisis it should be investigated.

## Fluid replacement

Fluid balance should be monitored and if oral intake is not adequate it should be supplemented with parenteral or nasogastric fluids. Cannulation of the leg veins should be avoided because of the risk of thrombosis and ulcers.

## Oxygen

Small trials have shown no benefit for routine use of oxygen. It should be given if pulse oximetry is below the patient's steady state. Some patients have low steady-state oxygen saturations but, if this is not known, then it is recommended that oxygen should be given when pulse oximetry is <95%.[1] It should be remembered that if a sickle cell patient has a

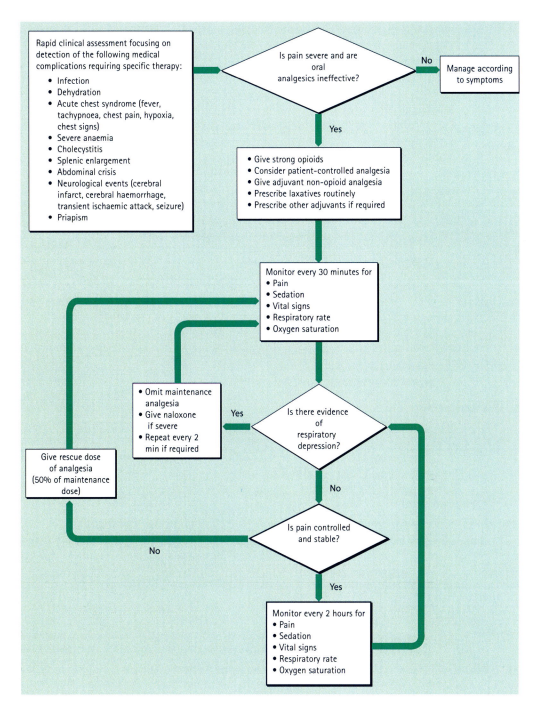

**Figure 10.1** Algorithm for the management of acute pain in opioid-naïve adults (adapted with permission from the British Committee for Standards in Haematology guidelines[1]).

low haemoglobin and increased methaemoglobin and carboxyhaemoglobin because of haemolysis, pulse oximetry will result in a higher haemoglobin oxygen saturation value than blood oximetry.

## Antibiotics

Due to hyposplenism and more subtle alterations in immunity, SCD patients are more susceptible to serious infection, especially *Streptococcus pneumoniae*, *Haemophilus influenzae B*, meningococcus and *Salmonella* species. Generally, the usual prophylactic antibiotics should be continued but it is recommended that broad-spectrum antibiotics should be started if the patient has a temperature of >38°C, is generally unwell, has chest symptoms or signs, or has other clinical evidence of infection.[1] The WBC count is often elevated in the steady state so this is not a reliable indicator of infection. If the patient is receiving iron chelation and has abdominal pain or diarrhoea, the chelation should be stopped, blood and stool cultures should be sent and ciprofloxacin should be started for possible *Yersinia* infections.

## Blood transfusion

In an uncomplicated painful crisis, haemoglobin may fall 1–2 g/dl and blood transfusion is not routinely indicated. Haemoglobin S has reduced oxygen affinity, thereby shifting the haemoglobin oxygen dissociation curve to the right, so symptoms of anaemia are usually mild. However, blood transfusion is indicated if there are signs or symptoms that may be due to anaemia and is more appropriate if there is a low reticulocyte count (<100 $\times 10^9$/l) and falling haemoglobin.[1]

If blood transfusion becomes necessary, the possibility of splenic or hepatic sequestration or parvovirus infection should be considered. The aim should be to return the haemoglobin to the steady-state level. Blood should be leukocyte depleted and matched for ABO, Rhesus (C, D and E) and Kell antigens.[4] Exchange transfusions are indicated for severe chest crises, suspected cerebrovasular events and multiorgan failure.[1] Sickle cell trait–negative blood should be used for exchange transfusions. Extended phenotype matching should be done for all patients with alloantibodies.[4]

## Physiotherapy

Incentive spirometry has been shown to be beneficial in patients with chest pain, back pain, chest infection or hypoxia, reducing the risk of acute chest syndrome (ACS) and atelectasis.[5]

## Acute chest syndrome

For the patient described above, the cause of his deterioration after admission is likely to be ACS.

Acute chest syndrome is a leading cause of death in adults with SCD. In a prospective multicentre study,[6] published in 2000, ACS was defined as the onset of new lobar infiltration on CXR and fever of over 38.5°C with tachypnoea and wheezing or cough. In this multicentre study the cause of ACS was not identified in about one-half of the 153 patients aged over 20 years. When the aetiology was identified, infection was the most common cause and included a substantial incidence of atypical organisms. However, about a quarter of those with known aetiology had fat embolism. About half of the patients were admitted for other reasons and developed ACS within 3 days. Those aged over 20 years were more likely to have complications and had a death rate of 9%.

| Table 10.1 Management of acute chest syndrome |
| --- |
| ● Oxygen supplementation to correct hypoxia |
| ● Respiratory therapy including use of incentive spirometry |
| ● Antibiotic therapy (including coverage for community-acquired and atypical pathogens) |
| ● Monitor intake and output: maintain euvolemia |
| ● Pain management: minimize chest splinting and avoid oversedation |
| ● Bronchodilator therapy if reactive airway disease (consider empiric trial in all patients) |
| ● Red blood cell transfusion if respiratory compromise or clinical deterioration* |

*If anaemia is significant, simple transfusion can be used, but exchange transfusion to decrease the HbS level to 30% or less should be considered if there is respiratory decompensation or other organ failure.[7]

A recent American Society of Hematology review of an evidence-based approach to the treatment of SCD[7] recommended management of ACS according to the treatment protocol of the National Acute Chest Syndrome Study Group (Table 10.1).

Data from the Cooperative Study of Sickle Cell Disease (CSSCD) showed that HbF levels were inversely related to the incidence of ACS[8] and to mortality.[9] Patients with ACS with HbF levels above the 75th percentile survived longer and an increase of HbF from 5% to 15% halved the incidence of ACS. High steady-state leukocyte count was also associated with higher ACS incidence and higher mortality.

The patient recovers and a few weeks later is seen in the outpatient clinic. Haemoglobin electrophoresis confirms the diagnosis of homozygous SCD.

**What is the management plan?**

Chronic problems associated with SCD can affect most systems and include:

- murmurs and tachycardia (anaemia), iron overload (if high transfusion requirement);
- pulmonary hypertension;
- gall stones secondary to chronic haemolysis (may be a cause of increased jaundice);
- renal papillary necrosis, inability to concentrate urine, enuresis, chronic renal failure, priapism;
- convulsions, transient ischaemic attacks and stroke;
- proliferative retinopathy, retinal artery occlusion, retinal detachment;
- avascular necrosis (femur and/or humerus), arthritis and osteomyelitis (*Salmonella* infection);
- leg ulceration – pathogenesis not elucidated but vaso-occlusion contributes to poor healing;
- repeated splenic infarction, which leads to hyposplenism, usually by 9–12 months, and subsequent susceptibility to infection;
- possible growth retardation and delayed sexual maturation.

Predictors of adverse outcomes indentified in the CSSCD are shown in Table 10.2.

| Table 10.2 Predictors of adverse outcomes indentified in the Cooperative Study of Sickle Cell Disease | |
|---|---|
| Predictors | Outcomes |
| ↓ Hb concentration | Death, stroke, leg ulcers |
| ≠ Hb concentration | Pain, ACS, AVN |
| ↓ HbF concentration | Death, ACS, pain, leg ulcers |
| ≠ Steady-state WBCs | Death, ACS |
| α-Thalassaemia present | AVN |
| α-Thalassaemia absent | Stroke |
| ≠ Pain rate | Adult death, AVN |
| Acute anaemia | Death, stroke |

ACS, acute chest syndrome; AVN, avascular necrosis; Hb, haemoglobin; WBC, white blood cells.

## Modifying factors

Observations that the onset of clinical manifestations of SCD are not apparent in the first few months of life until HbF levels fall and evidence that lower levels of HbF were associated with adverse outcomes (the CSSCD data) triggered the search for drugs that target the epigenetic silencing of fetal globin genes. A number of drugs have been shown to do this in animal models and patients. These include the DNA hypomethylating agents 5-azacytidine and decitabine, the histone deacetylase inhibitor butyrate, the ribonucleotide reductase inhibitor hydroxycarbamide (hydroxyurea [HU]) and erythropoietin.[10]

In 1995 the Multicenter Study of Hydroxyurea in Sickle Cell Anemia (MSH) was published.[11] This landmark study was a randomized, double-blind, placebo-controlled clinical trial to test the hypothesis that HU could substantially reduce the frequency of painful crises in adults with sickle cell anaemia. Patients with HbSS aged >18 years and experiencing three or more painful episodes per year were enrolled. The trial was stopped early because of beneficial effects in the treatment arm and subsequently led to US Food and Drug Administration approval for HU in SCD. In the MSH there was a 50% reduction in the incidence of ACS in the HU treatment group compared to the control group. Higher baseline HbF level predicted a better response in children but not adults. There was a variable response to HU and about one-third of patients did not respond. Toxicity associated with HU (bone marrow suppression) is reversible.

In the case of the patient described above, in addition to monitoring for the complications of SCD and ensuring compliance with prophylactic antibiotics and the recommended immunizations for hyposplenism, he should be given the option to start hydroxycarbamide. Improvement can be seen before there is a significant increase in HbF levels and it is postulated that a fall in WBC count may be partly responsible.

## Recent Developments

To date, the only curative treatment for SCD is haematopoietic stem cell transplantation. However, even if a donor can be found, the procedure is associated with significant morbidity and mortality and therefore only suitable for a few patients with severe disease. For the vast majority treatment is aimed at the management of crises and prevention of complications but new insights are being made into the pathophysiology of SCD and these are leading to new approaches to therapy. One of these is the concept that sickle cell complications form a spectrum of sub-phenotypes determined by haemolytic rate. These range from the viscosity-vaso-occlusion sub-phenotype, associated with a lower haemolytic rate, to the haemolysis-endothelial dysfunction sub-phenotype, which is associated with a higher haemolytic rate and consequent low nitric oxide bioavailability.[12] The former is associated with higher incidence of vaso-occlusive crises, acute chest syndrome and lower HbF levels. The latter is associated with a high prevalence of pulmonary hypertension, leg ulceration, priapism and stroke. Therapies which target the reduced nitric oxide bioavailability and vasculopathy are emerging. A number have been tested in humans and these include sildenafil, bosentan, arginine, glutamine and niacin.[12] Other developments include gene therapy which is entering phase I/II trials and therapies aimed at preventing red cell dehydration. It is likely that future treatments will combine agents with different pharmacological targets to maximize therapeutic effect and minimize side effects.

# Conclusion

In the 1960s and 1970s, SCD was thought to be a disease of childhood, with only a fraction of those affected living to adulthood. In one review in 1973 the median survival was 14.3 years. A third of patients died before the age of 5 years and only a sixth reached 30 years of age. More recently, in 1994, an estimate of median survival in the USA was 42 years for men and 48 years for women. In Jamaica in 2001, median survival was 53 years for men and 58.5 years for women. Thus, in the developed world there have been marked improvements in survival in SCD. ACS is a leading cause of death and the patient described in this chapter should benefit from the introduction of hydroxycarbamide into his care plan.

However, there are no firm data on the survival of patients with SCD on the African continent, where sickle cell anaemia contributes to 5% of deaths in children aged under 5 years.[2] This rises to 9% in West Africa and up to 15% in individual West African countries. In the developing world, malaria remains a major cause of ill health and death in children with sickle cell anaemia.[2] The very factor that is thought to be responsible for the positive selection of the sickle cell gene continues to influence the outcome and manifestations of sickle cell anaemia in Africa.

# Further Reading

1 Rees DC, Olujohungbe AD, Parker NE, Stephens AD, Telfer P, Wright J. Guidelines for the management of the acute painful crisis in sickle cell disease. *Br J Haematol* 2003; **120**: 744–52.

2 World Health Organization. *Sickle-cell anaemia*. Geneva: World Health Organization, 2006.

3 Benjamin LJ, Dampier CD, Jacox AK, *et al. Guideline for the Management of Acute and Chronic Pain in Sickle Cell Disease*. Glenview, IL: American Pain Society, 1999.

4  Vichinsky EP, Earles A, Johnson RA, Hoag MS, Williams A, Lubin B. Alloimmunization in sickle cell anemia and transfusion of racially unmatched blood. *N Engl J Med* 1990; **322**: 1617–21.

5  Bellet PS, Kalinyak KA, Shukla R, Gelfand MJ, Rucknagel DL. Incentive spirometry to prevent acute pulmonary complications in sickle cell diseases. *N Engl J Med* 1995; **333**: 699–703.

6  Vichinsky EP, Neumayr LD, Earles AN, *et al.* Causes and outcomes of the acute chest syndrome in sickle cell disease. National Acute Chest Syndrome Study Group. *N Engl J Med* 2000; **342**: 1855–65.

7  Lottenberg R, Hassell KL. An evidence-based approach to the treatment of adults with sickle cell disease. *Hematology Am Soc Hematol Educ Program* 2005; 58–65.

8  Castro O, Brambilla DJ, Thorington B, *et al.* The acute chest syndrome in sickle cell disease: incidence and risk factors. The Cooperative Study of Sickle Cell Disease. *Blood* 1994; **84**: 643–9.

9  Platt OS, Brambilla DJ, Rosse WF, *et al.* Mortality in sickle cell disease. Life expectancy and risk factors for early death. *N Engl J Med* 1994; **330**: 1639–44.

10  Fathalla H, Atweh GF. Induction of fetal hemoglobin in the treatment of sickle cell disease. *Hematology Am Soc Hematol Educ Program* 2006; 58–62.

11  Charache S, Terrin ML, Moore RD, *et al.* Effect of hydroxyurea on the frequency of painful crises in sickle cell anemia. Investigators of the Multicenter Study of Hydroxyurea in Sickle Cell Anemia. *N Engl J Med* 1995; **332**: 1317–22.

12  Morris CR. Mechanisms of vasculopathy in sickle cell disease and thalassemia. *Hematology Am Soc Hematol Educ Program* 2008; 177–85.

PROBLEM

# 11 β-Thalassaemia major

## Case History

 A 21-year-old woman who has recently emigrated from Pakistan is referred to your clinic. She is known to have β-thalassaemia major and has been receiving regular blood transfusions.

**How would you approach the initial assessment of this patient?**

# Background

β-Thalassaemia major is a genetic disorder of haemoglobin synthesis caused by mutations affecting both β-globin genes on chromosome 11. Reduced production of β-globin chains leads to an excess of α-globin, which precipitates in red cell precursors resulting in their premature destruction and ineffective haematopoiesis. α-Chain precipitation also interferes with the red cells' passage through the microcirculation, shortening their survival time. Raised erythropoietin drives haematopoietic expansion in the spleen and marrow while increased iron absorption from the gut results in damage to the heart, liver and endocrine system. β-Thalassaemia major describes those individuals with a severe phenotype for whom normal growth and development would be impossible without regular transfusion. Symptoms develop around the age of 6 months as the main haemoglobin switches from haemoglobin F (HbF) to HbA. The affected child will be pale and fail to thrive. Marrow expansion causes skull bossing, zygomatic enlargement ('mongoloid facies') and dental malocclusion. Growth is stunted and long bone thinning may result in spontaneous fractures. Increased red cell turnover and the resulting hypermetabolic state may cause fever, wasting, gout and folate deficiency. Liver cirrhosis and thrombocytopenia due to hypersplenism lead to a bleeding tendency. Untreated, death occurs from infection or heart failure, often before the age of 2 years.

Regular blood transfusion to maintain haemoglobin at >9.5–10 g/dl, usually every 3–4 weeks, will inhibit marrow and spleen expansion and, initially, allow normal growth and development. However, transfusion also results in progressive iron loading, leading to hypogonadotrophic hypogonadism, short stature, failure of menarche and infertility. Liver disease and endocrine disturbance such as hypothyroidism, diabetes, growth hormone deficiency and hypoparathyroidism may also occur. Cardiac failure or acute arrhythmias usually prove fatal in the second or third decade of life.

These complications are largely preventable through iron chelation. Desferrioxamine 20–50 mg/kg subcutaneously (SC) for 8–12 hours, 5–7 days per week, is usually commenced before serum ferritin is >1000 μg/l or liver iron is >7 mg/g dry weight, which generally occurs after the twelfth transfusion. Oral vitamin C 100–250 mg on days when chelation is given increases urinary iron excretion. Iron stores must be monitored during therapy as excess chelation leads to toxicity. The target serum ferritin is usually around 1000 μg/l, while levels persistently greater than 2500 μg/l predict cardiac complications and death. Over the last few decades, survival has progressively improved and in a recent long-term follow-up study, 65% of patients were alive aged 35 years.[1] However, the majority of deaths are still due to cardiac events, and poor compliance with chelation, which is a particular challenge during adolescence, is associated with worse survival.[1,2] Since the 1980s, children with a human leukocyte antigen (HLA)-matched sibling have also had the option of bone marrow transplantation, which may be curative and has a disease-free survival of around 70%–80%.[3] Splenectomy has been carried out in those with high transfusion requirements (>220 ml red cells/kg/year) but is less commonly required if an appropriate transfusion regimen has been received from an early age.[4]

Infection remains the second most common cause of death after heart disease. Various immune alterations such as decreased CD4:CD8 ratio and defective neutrophil chemotaxis are described. Although such alterations are poorly understood, iron overload must have a prominent role.[5] Infectious species with increased virulence in the presence of excess iron include *Yersinia enterocolitica*, *Klebsiella* species, *Escherichia coli*,

*Pseudomonas* and *Legionella*. *Yersinia* is associated with desferrioxamine treatment and may present with colitis, arthritis or sepsis. If suspected, chelation should be stopped and appropriate antibiotics, e.g. ciprofloxacin, commenced. Asplenic patients are at increased risk of sepsis from encapsulated bacteria and severe malaria. They require pneumococcal, *Haemophilus influenzae* type b and conjugated meningococcal C vaccinations, prophylactic penicillin V and malarial prophylaxis at time of risk. Those with indwelling lines for transfusion or chelation are additionally at risk of catheter-related infection and febrile illness should be treated promptly. Transfusion-transmitted infections include human immunodeficiency virus (HIV) and hepatitis B and C, which may lead to cirrhosis and secondary hepatocellular carcinoma.

## Assessment

The review of the patient should be at a centre with experience in managing patients with thalassaemia. Translation services should be available if required. The assessment aims to detect complications of the disease or its treatment. Medical history will establish details of prior transfusions (time of onset, reactions), chelation (frequency, dose, route) and surgery (e.g. splenectomy); also, time of onset of puberty, current medications and family history should be documented. Examination should identify evidence of heart failure, organomegaly, stigmata of chronic liver disease, leg ulcers, pubertal development, endocrinopathies, dental or facial problems. Baseline investigations include full blood count, blood film, haemoglobin electrophoresis (may be affected by recent transfusion), blood group, red cell phenotype and antibody screen, hepatitis and HIV serology, thyroid, liver and renal function, blood glucose, and bone and sex hormone assays. DNA analysis for $\alpha$- and $\beta$-globin genotype (predicts severity of the clinical phenotype) should be considered. A dual-energy X-ray absorptiometry (DEXA) scan, echocardiogram and T2* magnetic resonance imaging (MRI) scan should also be requested.

Referral to a fertility unit should be offered, in order to discuss treatment options. The patient should also be given the option of self-referral to a psychologist. Audiometry and ophthalmology reviews are required if the patient is receiving desferrioxamine or deferasirox. Initial investigations may indicate that endocrine or cardiology referrals are needed and hepatitis B vaccinations should be organized if the patient is non-immune. Genetic counselling will be required and social service review may be helpful. Contact numbers for the unit and local support groups should also be provided.

The patient has been receiving an appropriate dose of desferrioxamine in Pakistan but her initial serum ferritin was 4500 µg/l without evidence of infection or inflammation. She continues with regular transfusions and her dose of desferrioxamine is increased from 25 mg/kg to 40 mg/kg, 6 days per week. Despite this, her serum ferritin rises to 4730 µg/l over 6 months. Her cardiac T2* is reported at 7 ms.

**How would you manage her iron chelation?**

Two oral iron chelators, deferiprone and more recently deferasirox, are available. They have been recently reviewed[6] and their characteristics are summarized in Table 11.1. In a randomized, controlled trial, deferasirox at 20–30 mg/kg/day maintained or reduced hepatic iron as effectively as desferrioxamine. As well as continuous scavenging of non-transferrin-bound labile plasma iron, which is responsible for tissue damage, *in*

**Table 11.1** Comparison of chelating agents

| | Desferrioxamine | Deferiprone | Deferasirox |
|---|---|---|---|
| Administration | SC or IV | Oral | Oral (soluble tablets) |
| Plasma half-life | Short (minutes). SC infused for 8–12 hours, 5–7 days/week; IV continuous | Moderate (<2 hours). Taken three times daily | Long (8–16 hours). Taken once daily |
| Dose | SC: 20–50 mg/kg/day. IV: consider starting at 50 mg/kg/day, titrate to keep therapeutic index <0.025* | 75–100 mg/kg/day | 20–30 mg/kg/day |
| Iron excretion | Mainly urine | Mainly urine | Faeces |
| Important side effects | Invasive infections at needle or line sites. With excess chelation: high tone deafness, blurred vision, loss of light and colour sensation, bone changes and short stature | Gastrointestinal (14%), arthralgia/arthritis (9%), raised ALT (usually transient, 7%), neutropenia (6%), agranulocytosis (neutrophils <0.5 × 10⁹/l, 0.8%), zinc deficiency | Gastrointestinal (upper GI ulceration and haemorrhage reported), rash (11%), raised creatinine (dose dependent), renal tubulopathy, headache, hearing and visual disturbance, hepatic dysfunction |
| Cost | SC – Intermediate | Lowest | Highest |
| Efficacy | Effective in reducing iron stores. Continuous IV therapy effective in reversing symptomatic cardiac overload | Hepatic: may be less effective than SC desferrioxamine as a single agent. Cardiac: effective | Hepatic: as effective as SC desferrioxamine. Little long-term data. Cardiac: promising but more clinical data needed |
| Licence | Approval in EU and US for iron overload in thalassaemia | EU approval (2000) – in β-thalassaemia major for treatment of iron overload in patients for whom desferrioxamine is contraindicated or results in serious toxicity. Available in US on compassionate-use basis only. | EU approval (2006) – in β-thalassaemia major for transfusional iron overload in patients >5 years; also in those with infrequent blood transfusion or aged 2–5 years for whom desferrioxamine is inadequate. FDA approval (2005) for patients >2 years for transfusional iron overload |

*Therapeutic index = mean daily dose of desferrioxamine (mg/kg)/serum ferritin (μg/l). ALT, alanine transferase; EU, Europe; FDA, US Food and Drug Administration; GI, gastrointestinal; IV, intravenous; SC, subcutaneous.

*vitro* studies show that deferasirox has rapid access to the intracellular iron pools within cardiac myocytes. Initial clinical reports suggest that deferasirox can also reduce cardiac iron. An additional benefit is that adherence to chelation is better with this once-daily tablet compared to SC desferrioxamine. Deferiprone also appears to be an effective chelator of cardiac iron. Its molecular properties also allow it to reach intracellular iron and in a randomized trial of patients without symptomatic heart failure, those receiving deferiprone had significant improvements in T2* and left ventricular ejection fraction compared to those on SC desferrioxamine. An Italian cohort study noted no cardiac events in patients on deferiprone, unlike those on desferrioxamine, while the authors of a large Cypriot study suggested that the improved survival seen after 2000 may be due to the introduction of combination therapy with deferiprone and desferrioxamine.[6,7] Although effective at cardiac iron chelation, some studies suggest that deferiprone is less effective than desferrioxamine at removing hepatic iron.[8] The use of deferiprone daily combined with 2–6 days of subcutaneous desferrioxamine has been shown to reduce serum ferritin and hepatic iron concentration more than either agent alone. Combination therapy also improves cardiac function. The 'shuttle' hypothesis has been put forward, where deferiprone mobilizes intracellular iron, which is exchanged in the plasma to the higher-affinity desferrioxamine molecule and excreted in the urine. Combination therapy has the additional benefit of reducing the number of days that an infusion pump is required, which is likely to improve compliance. Conventional management of severe cardiac iron loading is by the use of a continuous intravenous (IV) desferrioxamine infusion through a central catheter. This has proven efficacy in reversing arrhythmias and heart failure.[9]

# Recent Developments

1 There is an increased risk of osteoporosis and patients are monitored with DEXA scanning. The cause appears to be multifactorial and bone marrow expansion, endocrine dysfunction, iron overload and genetic factors have important roles[10] While optimizing supportive care, patients are advised to exercise and increase dietary calcium and vitamin D intake, as well as to avoid smoking or excess alcohol. Hormone replacement therapy may be offered to those with hypogonadism and bisphosphonates to those with established osteoporosis.

2 Pythiosis, a rare aquatic, fungus-like infection caused by invasion of injured host tissue, is strongly associated with thalassaemia. Reported mainly in Asian patients, pythiosis may cause cutaneous granulomatous lesions, corneal ulcers and keratitis or cause gangrene or rupture of blood vessels. The latter is associated with high mortality. Medical treatment and antifungals are ineffective but a vaccine has been developed with therapeutic activity.[5]

3 Pregnancy with a successful outcome is now a realistic option. Some patients can conceive spontaneously, while those with hypogonadism may require induction of spermatogenesis or ovulation. There is a 30% increase in cardiac workload during pregnancy and a risk of accelerating cardiac dysfunction. Those with pre-existing cardiac disease are therefore advised not to undergo pregnancy.[11] Control of diabetes and thyroid function should be optimized, liver and cardiac function assessed and teratogenic medications – e.g. bisphosphonates, oral hypoglycaemics, angiotensin converting enzyme inhibitors and desferrioxamine – stopped. Red cell antibodies, rubella immune status and viral serology should be screened for, partner testing offered and folic acid prescribed. Calcium and vitamin D are required if pre-pregnancy bone density was reduced.

4 Ferritin is an acute-phase reactant and therefore serum ferritin is not always a reliable marker of iron stores. Liver iron concentration measured by tissue biopsy is invasive and can be inaccurate if the biopsy is small or cirrhosis is present. Magnetic resonance imaging is emerging as an effective, non-invasive alternative. Hepatic iron concentration measured by MRI R2 and R2* (the reciprocals of T2 and T2*, respectively) appears to correlate well with liver biopsy data.[12] Serum ferritin and liver biopsy appear to be inadequate as surrogate markers for cardiac iron, while cardiac dysfunction detectable on echocardiogram presents late.[13,14] Myocardial T2* directly reflects cardiac iron and correlates with left ventricular function,[13] appears reproducible between scanners[14] and should aid pre-symptomatic detection of cardiac iron, enabling earlier intensification of chelation

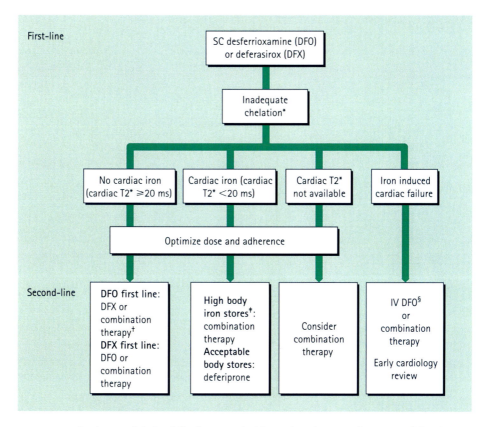

*Inadequate chelation defined as serum ferritin consistently greater than 1500 µg/l, liver iron >7 mg/g dry weight or cardiac T2* <20 ms.
†Combination therapy is SC DFO 40–50 mg/kg 2–5 days per week plus deferiprone 75–100 mg/kg/day 7 days per week.
‡High body iron stores defined as serum ferritin consistently greater than 1500 µg/l or liver iron >7 mg/g dry weight
§IV DFO delivered as a continuous infusion of 50–60 mg/kg/day via a port-a-cath.

**Figure 11.1** Approach to patients with an inadequate response to iron chelation therapy.

therapy. The lower limit of normal for cardiac T2* is 20 ms, while values <8 ms indicate severe iron loading.

5 Many patients do not have an HLA-matched sibling. In an Italian study of 68 patients undergoing bone marrow transplantation from matched unrelated donors, disease-free survival was 66% with chronic graft-versus-host disease in 18%.[15]

6 In 2005, the UK Thalassaemia Society issued standards for the delivery of clinical care, with performance indicators to provide quality assurance.[4] An updated second edition was published in 2008 (free to download at www.ukts.org/).[4]

## Conclusion

If there are symptoms or signs suggesting cardiac failure, the patient should be urgently refered to a cardiologist and chelation changed to continuous IV desferrioxamine or combination therapy. If there is no evidence of cardiac failure, issues of compliance must be explored. If adherence is a problem, it must be ensured that she understands the reasons for therapy and is able to set up infusions effectively. Disposable balloon pumps, home delivery and small 'thumb-tack' needles can help and psychological support may identify other barriers to compliance. If no treatable factors can be identified, an intensified form of chelation should be offered. Since she has both high total body iron stores (indicated by high ferritin) and severe cardiac iron loading, combination therapy would be the preferred option. Figure 11.1 illustrates an approach to the poorly chelated patient based on UK standards (Figure 11.1).[4]

## Further Reading

1 Borgna-Pignatti C, Cappellini MD, De Stefano P, *et al.* Survival and complications in thalassemia. *Ann N Y Acad Sci* 2005; **1054**: 40–47.

2 Modell B, Khan M, Darlison M. Survival in beta-thalassaemia major in the UK: data from the UK Thalassaemia Register. *Lancet* 2000; **355**: 2051–2.

3 Lawson SE, Roberts IA, Amrolia P, Dokal I, Szydlo R, Darbyshire PJ. Bone marrow transplantation for beta-thalassaemia major: the UK experience in two paediatric centres. *Br J Haematol* 2003; **120**: 289–95.

4 Yardumian A, Telfer P, Constantinou G, *et al.* Standards for the clinical care of children and adults with thalassaemia in the UK. www.ukts.org/. 2008.

5 Vento S, Cainelli F, Cesario F. Infections and thalassaemia. *Lancet Infect Dis* 2006; **6**: 226–33.

6 Neufeld EJ. Oral chelators deferasirox and deferiprone for transfusional iron overload in thalassemia major: new data, new questions. *Blood* 2006; **107**: 3436–41.

7 Telfer P, Coen PG, Christou S, *et al.* Survival of medically treated thalassemia patients in Cyprus. Trends and risk factors over the period 1980–2004. *Haematologica* 2006; **91**: 1187–92.

8 Caro J, Huybrechts KF, Green TC. Estimates of the effect on hepatic iron of oral deferiprone compared with subcutaneous desferrioxamine for treatment of iron overload in thalassemia major: a systematic review. *BMC Blood Disord* 2002; **2**: 4.

9 Davis BA, Porter JB. Long-term outcome of continuous 24-hour desferrioxamine infusion via indwelling intravenous catheters in high-risk beta-thalassemia. *Blood* 2000; **95**: 1229–36.

10 Voskaridou E, Anagnostopoulos A, Konstantopoulos K, *et al.* Zoledronic acid for the treatment of osteoporosis in patients with beta-thalassemia: results from a single-center, randomized, placebo-controlled trial. *Haematologica* 2006; **91**: 1193–202.

11 Tuck SM. Fertility and pregnancy in thalassemia major. *Ann N Y Acad Sci* 2005; **1054**: 300–307.

12  Wood JC, Enriquez C, Ghugre N, *et al*. MRI R2 and R2* mapping accurately estimates hepatic iron concentration in transfusion-dependent thalassemia and sickle cell disease patients. *Blood* 2005; **106**: 1460–65.

13  Pennell DJ. T2* magnetic resonance and myocardial iron in thalassemia. *Ann N Y Acad Sci* 2005; **1054**: 373–8.

14  Tanner MA, He T, Westwood MA, Firmin DN, Pennell DJ. Multi-center validation of the transferability of the magnetic resonance T2* technique for the quantification of tissue iron. *Haematologica* 2006; **91**: 1388–91.

15  La Nasa G, Argiolu F, Giardini C, *et al*. Unrelated bone marrow transplantation for beta-thalassemia patients: The experience of the Italian Bone Marrow Transplant Group. *Ann N Y Acad Sci* 2005; **1054**: 186–95.

# Clinical Blood Transfusion

## PROBLEM

# 12   Acute haemolytic transfusion reaction (ABO incompatibility)

## Case History

A 45-year-old woman with severe menorrhagia due to uterine fibroids has failed to respond to medical treatment and is admitted for elective abdominal hysterectomy. Her pre-operative blood count shows haemoglobin (Hb) 10.5 g/dl (reference range 11.5–16.5) and mean cell volume 75 fl (80–98). On the first post-operative day her Hb is 9.5 g/dl but pulse rate and blood pressure are normal. Her surgeon orders that she be transfused with two units of red cells. She has never been transfused before. Ten minutes after starting the first unit of red cells she complains of pain at the infusion site, rapidly followed by the onset of rigors, vomiting and bilateral loin pain. On examination she is flushed and agitated, and has pulse rate 140 beats/min, blood pressure 90/60 mmHg and temperature 37.5°C. Within minutes she becomes increasingly shocked and confused and blood starts oozing from her fresh abdominal wound. The urine in her urinary catheter bag is noted to be red.

What is the most likely cause of her acute deterioration?

What is the most important differential diagnosis?

How would you manage and investigate the problem?

What are the most likely root causes of this problem and what preventative measures can be taken?

# Background

The clinical picture in this case is highly suggestive of an acute haemolytic transfusion reaction, most likely caused by ABO incompatibility. The most important differential diagnosis is a reaction to a bacterially contaminated red cell unit.

The ABO blood group system, discovered by Landsteiner in 1901, is the most important in clinical transfusion practice. Reciprocal antibodies to the patient's A or B group are found in the plasma after the age of 4 to 6 months and are *naturally occurring* – i.e. they occur in the absence of immunization by transfusion or pregnancy (they are probably stimulated by ABO-like substances on colonic bacterial flora) (Table 12.1). These antibodies activate the complement cascade and cause intravascular haemolysis, with the potential to initiate disseminated intravascular coagulation (DIC) and a potentially fatal systemic inflammatory response.

Most fatal reactions occur when group O patients are inadvertently transfused with red cells of group A or B.

| Table 12.1 The ABO blood group system | | | |
|---|---|---|---|
| Blood group | Antigens on cells | Antibodies in serum | Proportion of UK donors |
| O | None | Anti-A + Anti-B | 47% |
| A | A | Anti-B | 42% |
| B | B | Anti-A | 8% |
| AB | A + B | None | 3% |

## Management and investigation

Acute haemolytic transfusion reactions are a medical emergency. Every hospital should have a clear written policy for the management and investigation of acute transfusion reactions (an example is given in Figure 12.1). It should be immediately available in clinical areas and all medical and nursing staff who administer or supervise transfusions should have appropriate training and competency assessment. Rapid recognition and early intervention are crucial in achieving a successful outcome. In most cases, symptoms and signs of a reaction begin soon after transfusion of the offending unit is commenced. Pulse rate, temperature and blood pressure should be recorded before the start of each unit and guidelines emphasize the critical importance of repeating the clinical observations 15 minutes into the transfusion episode, when most serious reactions will be evident. This check is crucial in anaesthetized or unconscious patients who are unable to report symptoms.

If a serious reaction is suspected, the transfusion must be stopped immediately, disconnected from the patient and venous access maintained with physiological saline. Urgent medical advice should be called. The details on the compatibility label on the unit of blood should be checked against the patient's identity bracelet and prescription and medical record. If possible, the patient's identity should be checked verbally. Any discrepancy should immediately be reported to the Blood Transfusion Laboratory so that the fate of the unit intended for the patient can be established (it may be at risk of being

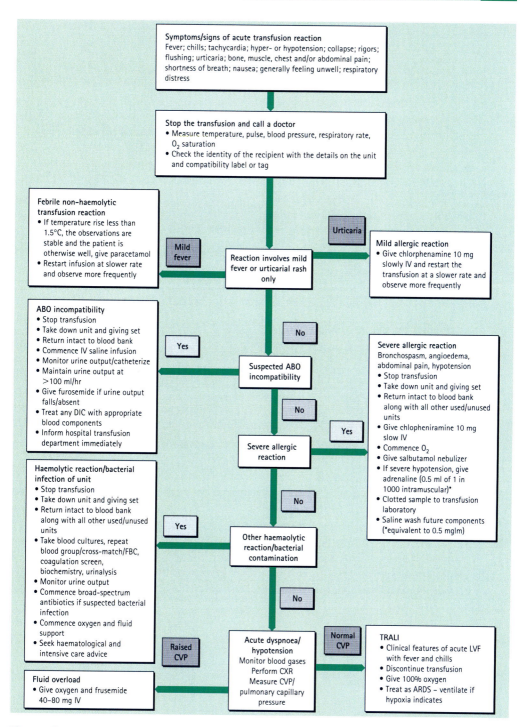

**Figure 12.1** Acute transfusion reactions (reproduced with permission from Dr DBL McClelland[1]). FBC, full blood count; CXR, chest X-ray; CVP, central venous pressure; LVF, left ventricular failure; ARDS, adult respiratory distress syndrome; TRALI, transfusion-related acute lung injury.

transfused to another patient). The blood bag and giving set must be returned intact to the laboratory and samples sent urgently for the following key investigations:

- repeat blood group, antibody screen and cross-match using pre- and post-transfusion blood samples and direct antiglobulin test (looking for antibodies on the post-transfusion red cells);
- evidence of red cell destruction (haemolysis – fall in Hb, spherocytes on the blood film, raised bilirubin and lactate dehydrogenase and haemoglobinuria [an indicator of intravascular haemolysis]);
- evidence of DIC – coagulation screen (prolonged prothrombin time [PT]/activated partial thromboplastin time [APTT]), low fibrinogen, raised D-dimer and fragmented red cells on blood film);
- evidence of renal dysfunction – renal function tests and electrolytes;
- blood cultures to exclude septicaemia from a bacterially contaminated unit.

It is crucial to involve medical staff of appropriate seniority at the earliest juncture. These are likely to include the haematologist, nephrologist and intensivist. In severe reactions, survival of the patient will depend on expert, rapid management of shock, renal dysfunction and coagulopathy.

### Root cause and prevention

Fatal acute haemolytic transfusion reactions due to ABO incompatibility between donor red cells and antibodies in the patient's plasma are estimated to occur in around 1 in every 600 000 transfusion episodes in developed countries. Most of these incidents are caused by clinical errors (failure of positive patient identification) at the time of pre-transfusion blood sampling (*wrong blood in tube*), collecting the wrong blood from the hospital blood bank or satellite refrigerator, or failure to perform the final bedside check correctly.[2] It has been estimated that around 1 in every 12 000 transfusions is given to the wrong recipient and 1 in every 2000 blood samples sent to a hospital laboratory is taken from the wrong patient.

It is important to analyse all serious adverse transfusion reactions in an open 'no blame' manner so that appropriate corrective actions can be taken (e.g. staff retraining, systems improvement). In this case history, the *root cause* of the episode can be traced back to the pre-operative assessment and management of the patient. Her blood picture is typical of chronic iron-deficiency anaemia, presumably due to menorrhagia, which should have been corrected with oral iron before surgery. The decision to transfuse a clinically and haemodynamically stable patient post-operatively at a Hb of 9.5 g/dl is contradicted by modern evidence-based clinical guidelines.[3,4]

## Recent Developments

Analysis of incidents reported to SHOT shows that most cases arise from misidentification errors at the time of blood sampling or collection of blood from the blood bank. Improved local policies and training have resulted in a significant reduction in the incidence of ABO haemolytic transfusion reactions in the UK, from 36 in 1997/98 to 10 in 2008 (with no deaths and one major morbidity). The use of electronic ID systems to identify patients, samples and components throughout the 'transfusion chain', as recommended by the National Patient Safety Agency, will help to eliminate human error.

# Conclusion

Initial investigations confirmed a fall in Hb compared with the pre-transfusion level with marked red cell fragmentation in the blood film. Coagulation tests confirmed DIC and intravascular haemolysis with haemoglobinuria. The patient went into acute renal failure despite prompt challenge with fluids and diuretics, and dialysis was required. Laboratory testing confirmed that this group O Rh(D)-negative patient had been transfused group A Rh(D)-negative red cells intended for another patient. Root-cause analysis established that the error had occurred when blood for another patient with a similar name was collected from the blood bank by the ward staff and the error was not identified at the bedside ID check. The patient survived.

# Further Reading

1 McClelland DBL (ed). *Handbook of Transfusion Medicine*, 4th edition. London: The Stationery Office, 2007. www.transfusionguidelines.org.uk

2 Serious Hazards of Transfusion (SHOT). *SHOT Report 2008*, 2008. www.shot-uk.org

3 British Committee for Standards in Haematology (BCSH). Guidelines for the administration of blood and blood components and the management of transfused patients, 1999. www.bcshguidelines.com

4 Scottish Intercollegiate Guidelines Network (SIGN). Perioperative blood transfusion for elective surgery. Clinical Guideline 54, 2001. www.sign.ac.uk

## PROBLEM

# 13 Massive blood transfusion

## Case History

A 36-year-old man is involved in a serious road traffic accident. On arrival at the emergency unit he is unconscious and shocked. After initial resuscitation, including the administration of physiological saline and synthetic colloids, X-rays and a computed tomography scan quickly establish that he has fractures of the right femur and pelvis, a right-sided haemothorax and haemoperitoneum with subdiaphragmatic gas. Baseline haematology (before transfusion) shows haemoglobin (Hb) 12.6 g/dl (reference range 13.5–18.0 g/dl) and platelets $140 \times 10^9/l$ ($150–400 \times 10^9/l$). A coagulation screen shows prothrombin time (PT) 15 seconds (control 12 seconds), activated partial thromboplastin time (APTT) 42 seconds (control 32 seconds) and fibrinogen 2.0 g/l (reference range 2.0–4.5 g/l). Laparotomy shows a ruptured spleen, jejunal transection and profuse bleeding. There are bilateral large subdural haematomas. Despite surgical intervention, the patient continues to bleed rapidly into the abdominal and chest cavities and, over the next 4 hours, he receives 20 units of red cells, two adult therapeutic doses (8 units) of platelets and 4 units of fresh frozen plasma. At this point he is oozing blood from previously haemostatic surgical wounds and intravenous catheter sites, systolic blood pressure is falling again and urine output is decreasing. Repeat blood tests show Hb 6.3 g/dl, white blood cells $5.0 \times 10^9/l$, platelets $50 \times 10^9/l$, PT 25 seconds, APTT 64 seconds and fibrinogen 0.8 g/l. A blood film is reported as showing fragmented red cells.

**What is your interpretation of the haematological and coagulation changes described above?**

**How would you define massive blood loss?**

**What are the key features of a massive blood loss protocol and of the management of the associated haematological problems?**

## Background

On arrival at the emergency unit the patient has a near-normal Hb concentration. However, in the early stages of major acute haemorrhage, the Hb concentration and haematocrit give a poor indication of the degree of blood loss because of haemoconcentration and peripheral vasoconstriction. Both the PT and APTT are only slightly prolonged but, of note, the fibrinogen concentration is at the low limit of normal.

Fibrinogen is an acute-phase reactant protein and one would expect the level to be markedly elevated in a patient with severe tissue injury. This, taken together with the slight thrombocytopenia, suggests that excessive consumption of clotting factors and platelets is already occurring.

By the time the blood tests are repeated, there is marked prolongation of PT and APTT and significant thrombocytopenia and hypofibrinogenaemia. The presence of fragmented red cells in the blood film and the clinical picture of generalized bleeding are indicative of disseminated intravascular coagulation (DIC).

## Management of massive blood loss and transfusion

Massive blood loss is defined as the loss of more than one blood volume within 24 hours (around 70 ml/kg, or 5 litres in a 70 kg adult), 50% of total blood volume lost in less than 3 hours or a rate of bleeding in excess of 150 ml/min. Early recognition and intervention is essential. The immediate priorities are to restore or maintain tissue perfusion and oxygenation to prevent irreversible vital organ damage followed by achieving control of the cause of bleeding. Massive haemorrhage associated with major trauma or obstetric emergencies is often associated with early activation of the coagulation and fibrinolytic systems, leading to DIC. Patients with the 'lethal triad' of acidosis, hypothermia and coagulopathy have a high mortality. Hypothermia reduces the activity of many clotting factors. In major sustained bleeding after surgery, dilution of clotting factors by massive transfusion is often the primary cause of bleeding. Successful management demands a protocol-driven multidisciplinary team approach and involvement of medical and surgical staff of sufficient seniority and experience, underpinned by clear lines of communication between clinicians and the transfusion laboratory.[1] In an emergency situation it is essential to ensure correct transfusion identification procedures are performed and that an accurate record is kept of all blood components transfused. Regular 'fire drills' to test the protocol are important. An example of a protocol is shown in Table 13.1.

Blood component therapy is based on frequent monitoring of haematological and coagulation parameters, repeated after each intervention. Near-patient tests, such as thromboelastography, can be used to guide component therapy but require appropriate expertise in interpretation.[2]

**Red cell** transfusion is usually necessary if 30%–40% of total blood volume is lost and >40% loss is immediately life threatening. In extreme emergency, it may be necessary to transfuse group O red cells (females less than 50 years of age should receive Rhesus D negative to avoid sensitization). ABO group-specific red cells can be issued within 10 minutes of a sample arriving in the transfusion laboratory and the use of large volumes of group O blood, a scarce resource, should be avoided. Fully cross-matched blood is available in 30 to 40 minutes. Intra-operative cell-salvage devices may reduce the need for donor red cells in appropriate cases.

**Platelet** transfusion should be given to maintain the count above $50 \times 10^9/l$ in the bleeding patient (the platelet count predicted when two blood volumes have been replaced by red cell and plasma components; sooner if DIC is present).[3] Recent guidelines[1] recommend ordering platelets at a 'trigger' of $75 \times 10^9/l$ to compensate for delays in procuring the component from the blood centre. A platelet count of $100 \times 10^9/l$ may be an appropriate target for patients with high-velocity multiple trauma or central nervous system injury. One or two 'adult therapeutic doses' (equivalent to 4 or 8 units) should be transfused.

**Table 13.1 Example of a major haemorrhage protocol (adapted from *Handbook of Transfusion Medicine*, 4th edition,[5] with permission of the editor).**

| Objective | Action | Notes |
|---|---|---|
| Control the bleeding | Early intervention – surgical, endoscopic, radiological | Interventional radiography can be life saving |
| Restore circulating volume<br><br>In patients with major vessel or cardiac injury it may be appropriate to restrict volume replacement after discussion with surgical team | Insert wide-bore peripheral cannulae<br><br>Give adequate volumes of crystalloid/colloid/blood<br><br>Aim to maintain normal blood pressure and urine output >30 ml/hr (5 ml/kg/hr) | Blood loss is often underestimated<br><br>Refer to local guidelines for resuscitation of trauma patients and red cell transfusion<br><br>Monitor arterial pressure and CVP if unstable |
| Avoid exacerbating coagulation problems | Keep the patient warm | Warmed fluids  Space blankets |
| Use laboratory data to guide management | *Request laboratory tests:*<br><br>FBC, PT, APTT, fibrinogen, transfusion sample, biochemistry, blood gases<br><br>Repeat FBC, PT, APTT, fibrinogen every 4 hours or after 1/3 blood volume replacement or after infusion of FFP | Colloid solutions can prolong clotting times and interfere with blood grouping<br><br>Take samples early<br><br>FFP and platelets may be needed before tests results available |
| Have blood components available when needed | Request red cells<br><br>Pack volumes range from 180 to 350 ml<br><br>*Platelets needed?*<br><br>Anticipate count <50 x 109/l after 1.5–2.0 blood volume replacement<br><br>Dose: 1 or 2 'adult therapeutic doses'<br><br>*FFP needed?*<br><br>Anticipate coagulation factor deficiency after 1.0–1.5 blood volume replacement<br><br>Aim for PT and APTT <1.5 x control, fibrinogen >1.0 g/l<br><br>Allow for 30 min thaw time<br><br>Dose: 15–20 ml/kg (at least 1000 ml [4 units] in adult<br><br>*Cryoprecipitate needed?*<br><br>To replace fibrinogen and FVIIIc<br><br>Aim for fibrinogen >1.0g/l<br><br>Allow for 30 min thaw time<br><br>Dose: 2 x 5 unit donation pools for average adult | Rh D–positive red cells may be used in males and post-menopausal females in an emergency<br><br>Use blood warmer<br><br>Consider cell salvage<br><br>Target platelet count:<br><br>>100 x 109/l in multiple/CNS trauma<br><br>>75 x 109/l in other cases<br><br>PT and APTT >1.5 x mean control value correlates with increased surgical bleeding<br><br>May need to use FFP before test results available, but take sample for PT, APTT and fibrinogen before FFP transfused<br><br>Fibrinogen <0.5g/l associated with microvascular bleeding<br><br>Low fibrinogen prolongs all clotting times (PT and APTT) |
| Recognize and act on complications | Suspect DIC<br><br>Treat underlying cause | Shock, hypothermia and acidosis increase the risk of coagulation problems and are associated with worse outcomes |
| Manage intractable non-surgical bleeding | Consider the use of pharmacological agents:<br><br>tranexamic acid or aprotinin<br><br>recombinant activated factor VIIa | Some evidence aprotinin may exacerbate renal damage<br><br>rFVIIa is not licensed for this indication |

APTT, activated partial thromboplastin time; CNS, central nervous system; CVP, central venous pressure; FBC, full blood count; FFP, fresh frozen plasma; PT, prothrombin time.

**Fresh frozen plasma** is infused in doses of 15 to 20 ml/kg to maintain the PT and APTT at <1.5 times the mean normal value in bleeding patients (routinely seen after 150% blood volume replacement). Fresh frozen plasma is also a source of fibrinogen (target >1.0 g/l), although volume considerations may predicate the use of pooled cryoprecipitate. Therapy is guided by frequent coagulation testing and clinical response.

**Pharmacological agents** such as antifibrinolytics (e.g. tranexamic acid) may be useful in massive haemorrhage, although good clinical evidence for their use is lacking. Recombinant activated factor VII (rFVIIa) has been widely used 'off license' as a 'universal haemostatic agent'. The evidence for benefit remains largely anecdotal and good clinical trials of this expensive agent are urgently needed.[4, 5] Its use should be considered if bleeding continues despite adequate component replacement therapy and surgical or interventional radiology intervention, and all use should be audited. It is less effective in acidotic patients and survival depends on the severity of the underlying injuries. The increased risk of using rFVIIa has been confirmed by meta-analysis of placebo-controlled trials and an amendment of the Summary of Product Characteristics in June 2009 advises it should not be used outside the approved indications.

## Recent Developments

Recent experience in military trauma suggests that a more aggressive approach to early, *pre-emptive*, platelet and plasma replacement therapy, as part of 'damage control resuscitation'[6] may improve survival by prevention and reversal of coagulopathy. Red cells, FFP and platelets are given in a 1:1:1 ratio (this approach has still to be tested in randomized controlled trials but is supported by large retrospective audits).[7] Once patients are stabilised in intensive care, a restrictive approach to blood component transfusion is associated with reduced mortality from infection and lung injury.

## Conclusion

With the judicious use of blood products along the principles described above, the patient's condition stabilized in theatre allowing surgery to be completed with splenectomy and jejunal repair. Post-operatively the patient continued to ooze from drain sites but blood loss reduced slowly over the next 48 hours, with recovery of platelet count and normalization of coagulation tests. Recombinant activated factor VII was not used.

## Further Reading

1 British Committee for Standards in Haematology. Guidelines on the management of massive blood loss. *Br J Haematol* 2006; **135**: 634–41. www.bcshguidelines.com

2 Samama CM, Ozier Y. Near-patient testing of haemostasis in the operating theatre: an approach to appropriate use of blood in surgery. *Vox Sang* 2003; **84**: 251–5.

3 British Committee for Standards in Haematology. Guidelines for the use of platelet transfusions. *Br J Haematol* 2003; **122**: 10–23. www.bcshguidelines.com

4 Levi M, Peters M, Büller HR. Efficacy and safety of recombinant factor VIIa for treatment of severe bleeding: a systematic review. *Crit Care Med* 2005; **33**: 883–90.

5 McClelland DBL (ed). *Handbook of Transfusion Medicine*, 4th edition. London: The Stationery Office, 2007. www.transfusionguidelines.org.uk

6 Jansen JO, Thomas R, Loudon A, Brooks A. Damage control resuscitation for patients with major trauma. *Br Med J* 2009;**338**:b1778,doi 10.1136/bmj.b1778 (published 5 June 2009).

7 Rose AH, Kotze A, Doolan D, Norfolk DR, Bellamy MC. Massive transfusion – evaluation of current clinical practice and outcome in two large teaching hospital trusts in Northern England. *Vox Sanguinis* 2009; **97**: 247–53.

**PROBLEM**

# 14 Refractoriness to platelet transfusion

## Case History

A 55-year-old woman, with a history of pregnancies 30 and 25 years ago, is undergoing her second cycle of consolidation chemotherapy for acute myeloid leukaemia. By the seventh day after completing the cycle, her morning platelet count has been below $10 \times 10^9/l$ for ten days. Despite daily prophylactic platelet transfusions she has developed a widespread purpuric rash on her legs and trunk, blood blisters on the oral mucosa and recurrent episodes of epistaxis severe enough to need nasal packing. She has been febrile for seven days despite intravenous broad-spectrum antibiotic therapy. Repeated blood cultures are negative and she was started on intravenous amphotericin B two days ago. Her platelet count before the latest transfusion is $3 \times 10^9/l$. The platelet count is $5 \times 10^9/l$ one hour after transfusion of one adult therapeutic dose (4 units) of platelets and $3 \times 10^9/l$ 18 hours after the transfusion.

**What are the most likely causes of her failure to respond to platelet transfusions?**

**What investigations would you perform?**

**How would you manage her bleeding problem?**

## Background

It is standard practice in haematology units to give prophylactic platelet transfusions to patients with temporary bone marrow suppression after chemotherapy when their count falls below a predetermined trigger level, commonly $10 \times 10^9/l$.[1] It is important to note that the effectiveness of *prophylactic*, as opposed to *therapeutic* (i.e. to treat bleeding episodes), platelet transfusions in this setting has not been established by randomized controlled trials.[2]

Refractoriness to platelet transfusions is defined as the repeated failure to obtain a satisfactory response to platelet transfusions.[1] Although the response of a bleeding episode to transfusion of platelets is the most clinically relevant marker, it is usual to assess the response to prophylactic platelet transfusions by measuring the increase in platelet count in response to the transfusion. To standardize the response in terms of the patient's size and the dose of platelets transfused, formulae such as *platelet recovery* and *corrected count increment* have been derived. However, these are of limited value in routine clinical practice as they require knowledge of the precise platelet content in each unit transfused. Simpler indicators, such as failure of the 1-hour platelet increment to exceed the 'transfusion trigger' or a rise of less than $10 \times 10^9/l$ after 20 to 24 hours, can be used as measures of unsatisfactory response. Because the response to individual platelet transfusions is variable, the diagnosis of refractoriness should only be made after an unsatisfactory response to two or more transfusions.

Historically, platelet refractoriness has been reported in more than 50% of patients receiving repeated transfusions and the causes can be categorized as immune or non-immune. The non-immune causes are associated with increased platelet consumption, often related to infection and its treatment, and constitute the large majority of cases in current practice (Table 14.1).

| Table 14.1 Causes of non-immune platelet refractoriness |
| --- |
| Infection |
| Antibiotics – especially amphotericin B, possibly fluoroquinolones |
| Splenomegaly/hypersplenism |
| Disseminated intravascular coagulation (DIC) |
| Bleeding |

Human leukocyte antigen (HLA) alloimmunization is the most common cause of immune platelet refractoriness (Table 14.2) and its incidence depends on:

- previous sensitization to foreign HLA antigens (pregnancy, transfusion);
- the type of blood product transfused (the incidence has fallen significantly with the introduction of leukocyte depletion);
- the immunosuppressive effect of the disease and its treatment (it is more common in aplastic anaemia than acute myeloid leukaemia).

Primary HLA alloimmunization requires exposure to donor cells, such as lymphocytes, exhibiting both class I and class II HLA antigens together with antigen-presenting cells (e.g. dendritic cells) of donor origin. As platelets express only class I HLA antigens, leukocyte-depleted products are unlikely to cause primary alloimmunization. However, class I antigens are able to initiate a secondary immune response in pre-sensitized individuals. Therefore, the typical patient who now develops alloimmune refractoriness to 'random donor' platelet transfusion is a female sensitized by previous pregnancy. A randomized trial of 530 patients with acute leukaemia found an HLA-alloimmunization rate of 62% in those patients with previous pregnancies receiving non-leukocyte-depleted

| Table 14.2 Causes of immune platelet refractoriness |
| --- |
| Antibodies to antigens on platelets: |
|   HLA |
|   HPA |
|   ABO |
| Drug-dependent platelet antibodies |
| Platelet autoantibodies |
| Immune complexes |

products compared to 33% in those with no history of pregnancy.[3] Modern studies using pre-storage leukocyte-depleted products show a rate of primary sensitization of <3%. Other immune causes of platelet refractoriness, such as alloimmunization to human platelet antigens (HPA) or the presence of autoantibodies, are much less common but their identification may lead to clinically important changes in management.

Patients with platelet refractoriness should be investigated and managed according to the algorithm below (Figure 14.1).

If there are clinical factors likely to cause non-immune platelet refractoriness (most commonly sepsis) these should be treated vigorously and platelet transfusion from random donors continued. In the presence of bleeding, a higher dose or more frequent platelet transfusion may be helpful.

If a poor clinical or haematological response persists, or a non-immune cause seems unlikely, the patient should be screened by a specialist laboratory for the presence of HLA antibodies (usually by lymphocytotoxicity and enzyme immunoassay tests). Antibodies should be typed for specificity to help in the selection of compatible platelet donors (although broad-spectrum 'multispecific' HLA antibodies are often present in this setting). The presence of HLA antibodies is not proof of immune platelet refractoriness but the response to platelet transfusion from donors matched, as closely as possible, for the patient's HLA-A and HLA-B antigens should be assessed. ABO-compatible platelets should be used wherever possible and all HLA-matched platelet transfusions should be gamma-irradiated to prevent transfusion-associated graft-versus-host disease. In the UK, HLA-typed platelet donors can be selected from regional and national panels and donations are made by plateletpheresis. If there is a good response to HLA-matched platelets, transfusions should be continued, providing enough compatible donors are available. HLA antibodies reduce or disappear over time in a significant number of patients and it is helpful to repeat the HLA-antibody screen monthly during treatment. If there is no response to HLA-matched platelets it is reasonable to screen for HPA and other less common antibodies and reconsider the possibility of non-immune platelet refractoriness. Advice from a specialist in transfusion medicine should be sought.

# Recent Developments

 Universal prestorage leucodepletion of blood components in the UK to $<1 \times 10^6$ per pack (as a variant Creutzfeldt Jacob Disease [vCJD] risk reduction measure) has markedly

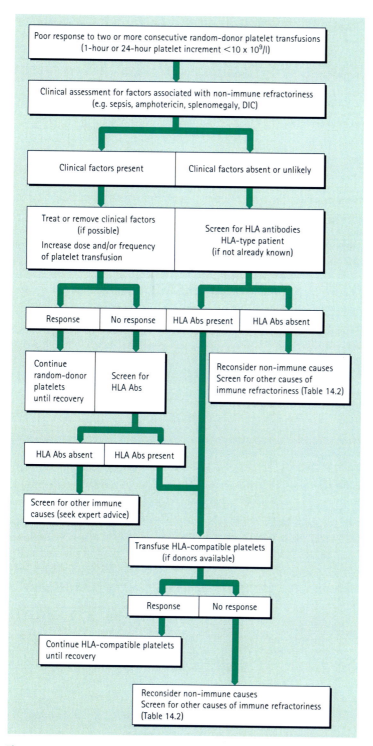

**Figure 14.1** Algorithm for diagnosing and treating refractoriness to platelet transfusion. Abs, antibodies; DIC, disseminated intravascular coagulation; HLA, human leukocyte antigen.

reduced the incidence of HLA immunisation in multi-transfused patients. A policy of therapeutic, as opposed to prophylactic platelet transfusion in haemato-oncology patients is being tested in a large multicentre randomized controlled trial in the UK (Trial of Platelet Prophylaxis – TOPPS) sponsored by NHS Blood and Transplant. Efforts to develop artificial platelets, for example freeze dried platelet membranes or 'synthocytes' (fibrinogen-coated albumin microspheres) have shown promise in animal models but none appears to be close to clinical development.

## Conclusion

The patient has several factors associated with a refractoriness to platelet transfusion. She has a probable infection and is receiving intravenous amphotericin B. However, she is a parous female, which significantly increases the probability of immune platelet refractoriness. In view of her bleeding, she should immediately be given a higher dose of random-donor platelets (e.g. two adult therapeutic doses) and the clinical and haematological response assessed. If the response is still unsatisfactory she should be screened for HLA antibodies. While the result is awaited it is reasonable to continue with high-dose random-donor platelets, ensuring they are ABO compatible and preferably less than 3 days old. If HLA antibodies are present, the most compatible donors should be identified and transfusion arranged. Post-transfusion (1 hour and 20–24 hour) platelet increments should be measured to assess the effectiveness of this treatment. Failure to respond clinically or haematologically should lead to further investigation and management according to the algorithm.

## Further Reading

1 British Committee for Standards in Haematology, Blood Transfusion Task Force. Guidelines for the use of platelet transfusions. *Br J Haematol* 2003; **122**: 10–23.

2 Stanworth SJ, Hyde C, Heddle N, Rebulla P, Brunskill S, Murphy MF. Prophylactic platelet transfusion for haemorrhage after chemotherapy and stem cell transplantation. *Cochrane Database Syst Rev* 2004; (4): CD004269.

3 The Trial to Reduce Alloimmunization to Platelets Study Group. Leukocyte reduction and ultraviolet B irradiation of platelets to prevent alloimmunization and refractoriness to platelet transfusion. *N Engl J Med* 1997; **337**: 1861–9.

# 15 Transfusion–related acute lung injury

## Case History

A previously healthy 45-year-old 80 kg man is admitted for an elective percutaneous liver biopsy under local anaesthetic as part of the investigation of probable genetic haemochromatosis diagnosed as part of a family study (plasma ferritin 1500 µg/l, C282Y homozygote). Pre-biopsy blood tests show a normal full blood count, slightly elevated alanine aminotransferase and a prothrombin time (PT) of 16 seconds (normal control 12 seconds). He is transfused with two units (approximately 500 ml) of fresh frozen plasma (FFP) 30 minutes before the biopsy 'to cover the procedure'. The biopsy goes ahead uneventfully. However, 90 minutes afterwards he complains of breathlessness, which becomes progressively worse during the next hour. On examination he is severely dyspnoeic at rest and centrally cyanosed. He has a tachycardia of 150 beats per minute, blood pressure 110/65 mmHg, temperature 38°C, no elevation of jugular venous pressure (JVP) and no peripheral oedema. Blood gases show severe hypoxia and hypocapnia. Chest X-ray (Figure 15.1) reveals a normal-sized heart but there is diffuse bilateral nodular and perihilar shadowing in the mid and lower zones of both lungs. His blood count is normal except for neutropenia ($1.2 \times 10^9$/l). He has no skin rashes or peripheral oedema.

**What is the most likely diagnosis?**

**How should the patient be treated?**

**How would you investigate the incident?**

**What measures can be taken to reduce the risk of this problem?**

## Background

The clinical picture is highly suggestive of transfusion-related acute lung injury (TRALI), indicated by the temporal relationship to transfusion, normal JVP, hypotension and acute neutropenia. Differential diagnosis would include left ventricular failure (LVF) precipitated by fluid overload – now known as transfusion associated circulatory over-load (TACO), (but there is no history of cardiac disease) or an acute allergic reaction (but there are no rashes or swelling).

Transfusion-related acute lung injury is a potentially life-threatening complication of blood transfusion most often, but not exclusively, related to the transfusion of plasma-

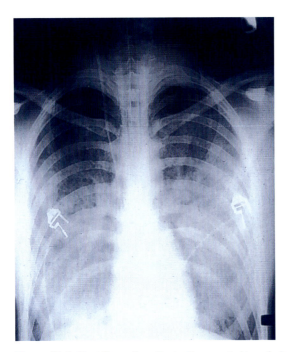

**Figure 15.1** Chest X-ray of a patient with suspected transfusion-related acute lung injury.

rich components such as FFP or platelets. It is a form of non-cardiogenic pulmonary oedema, clinically indistinguishable from acute respiratory distress syndrome, and is usually caused by the interaction of specific leukocyte antibodies in the transfused plasma with the patient's leukocytes. Antibodies to human leukocyte antigens (HLA class I or II) or human neutrophil antigens (HNA) are most often implicated.[1] HLA antibodies are found in up to 15% of multiparous female blood donors. Fatal cases of TRALI show an intense acute inflammatory infiltrate of neutrophils and monocytes in the alveolar spaces.[2] Activated leukocytes adhere to, or become trapped in, the pulmonary vasculature where the release of inflammatory mediators causes capillary leak and pulmonary oedema. Most patients receiving components from donors with HLA antibodies do not develop TRALI and there may be a need for a 'second hit' for it to occur.[3] 'Priming' and 'activating' factors in the patient may include recent surgery, hypoxia, trauma, sepsis or biologically active lipids in stored blood components.

Symptoms classically occur within 6 hours of transfusion but may occiasionally be delayed for up to 24 hours. Typical symptoms and signs include dyspnoea, cyanosis, hypotension and fever. Chest X-ray shows bilateral diffuse and nodular shadowing in the lungs, maximal in the mid and lower zones and perihilar areas. Left atrial pressure is usually normal or low in TRALI, in contrast to TACO. A low partial pressure of arterial oxygen/fraction of inspired oxygen ratio ($PaO_2/FiO_2$ Index <200) may also be helpful in distinguishing TRALI from TACO.[1] Transient neutropenia and/or monocytopenia are common at the start of the reaction, followed by neutrophil leucocytosis. The diagnosis of TRALI is based on the clinical picture but may later be supported by finding leukocyte antibodies in the donor plasma. Transfusion should be stopped immediately and treatment is primarily supportive until the lung injury subsides. There is a spectrum of severity, from mild pulmonary dysfunction to fatal respiratory failure. Severe cases may need mechanical ventilation and oxygen for several days but the prognosis for full recovery is good. There is no evidence that steroids are beneficial and inappropriate diuretic treatment, based on a misdiagnosis of LVF/TACO, may increase mortality. Suspected cases should immediately be reported to the hospital transfusion team or transfusion medicine specialist and the likelihood of TRALI assessed. Blood samples will be taken from the patient for HLA or HNA typing and the investigation coordinated with the transfusion service. Donors of components transfused within 24 hours of the reaction will be identified and screened for leukocyte antibodies according to a defined protocol (prioritizing investigation of female donors of plasma-rich components). The finding of a donor with an antibody reacting with the patient's leukocytes increases the probability that this case was TRALI. Donors implicated in 'highly likely' TRALI episodes may be resigned from the panel. Some cases of TRALI appear to be 'non-immune'; they tend to be milder and have been associated particularly with haematological malignancies and cardiac disease.

Clinical recognition of TRALI is often poor, but data from haemovigilance schemes and institutional surveys suggest that immune-mediated TRALI has an incidence of around 1 in 5000 units transfused and may be the most common cause of transfusion-related death in developed countries.

# Recent Developments

Reports by the UK Serious Hazards of Transfusion (SHOT) haemovigilance scheme[4] have confirmed the increased risk of TRALI with plasma-rich blood components, especially from female donors. In 2004, the UK Transfusion Services prioritized the

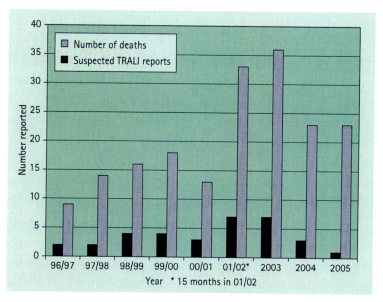

**Figure 15.2** Deaths at least possibly due to TRALI and number of reports of suspected TRALI by year. Data shown are from the annual SHOT Report 2007.[4]

production of FFP from male donors and this was followed by a significant fall in reports of, and deaths from, TRALI reported to SHOT (Figure 15.2).[4] Seventeen cases of probable TRALI were reported to SHOT in 2008 but there were no deaths. Transfusion-related acute lung injury has not been reported after infusion of solvent/detergent-treated plasma, probably because any leukocyte antibodies are diluted when plasma from many donors is pooled during production of this product.

Recent data suggests that transfusion of plasma-rich blood components may also be an important risk factor for increased morbidity and mortality from acute lung injury ('non-immune TRALI') in critically ill patients of many types.[7]

## Conclusion

The patient was admitted to the intensive therapy unit for oxygen therapy but subsequently deteriorated. Pulmonary artery pressure monitoring showed no evidence of LVF. The patient was intubated and ventilated for 48 hours, following which he made a full recovery. Subsequent investigation of the plasma donor confirmed the presence of leukocyte antibodies. Review of the case led to a change in policy regarding the use of FFP in the unit as regards liver biopsy. The most effective way to prevent TRALI, and other serious reactions, is to avoid unnecessary transfusions. The evidence base for much FFP transfusion is poor.[5] Although it is common practice to give *prophylactic* FFP before liver biopsy, there is little evidence that modest pre-procedure elevation of PT predicts an increased bleeding risk.[6] In any event, 2 units of FFP (around 500 ml) is no more than half the recommended therapeutic dose (15–20 ml/kg, 4 to 6 units) for an 80 kg man.

## Further Reading

1 Kleinman S, Caulfield T, Chan P, *et al.* Toward an understanding of transfusion-related acute lung injury: statement of a consensus panel. *Transfusion* 2004; **44**: 1774–89.

2 Wyncoll DL, Evans TW. Acute respiratory distress syndrome. *Lancet* 1999; **354**: 497–501.

3 Silliman CC. Transfusion-related acute lung injury. *Transfus Med Rev* 1999; **13**: 177–86.

4 Serious Hazards of Transfusion (SHOT). *SHOT Report 2007*, 2007. www.shot-uk.org

5 British Committee for Standards in Haematology. Guidelines for the use of fresh frozen plasma, cryoprecipitate and cryosupernatant. *Br J Haematol* 2004; **126**: 11–28.

6 Segal JB, Dzik WH. Paucity of studies to support that abnormal coagulation test results predict bleeding in the setting of invasive procedures: an evidence-based review. *Transfusion* 2005; **45**: 1413–25.

7 Benson AB, Moss M, Silliman C. Transfusion-related acute lung injury (TRALI): a clinical review with emphasis on the critically ill. *Br J Haematol* 2009; **147**: 431–3.

# Acute and Chronic Leukaemia and Myelodysplasia

**PROBLEM**

# 16  Acute myeloid leukaemia

## Case History

A 35-year-old female presented with fatigue and gum bleeding. On examination, gum hypertrophy with bleeding and splenomegaly were noted. A full blood count revealed a haemoglobin concentration of 8 g/dl, white cell count $120 \times 10^9$/l and platelets $15 \times 10^9$/l. Peripheral blood leukocytes were 90% myelomonocytic blasts. Bone marrow flow cytometry was CD34− CD33+ CD14+ CD56+ and karyotype was normal.

**How would this patient's 'risk' be assessed from the above information?**

**Would molecular studies reveal further prognostic markers?**

## Background

The survival for younger patients with acute myeloid leukaemia (AML) is improving decade on decade (Figure 16.1). It is now realistic to attempt curative therapy in almost

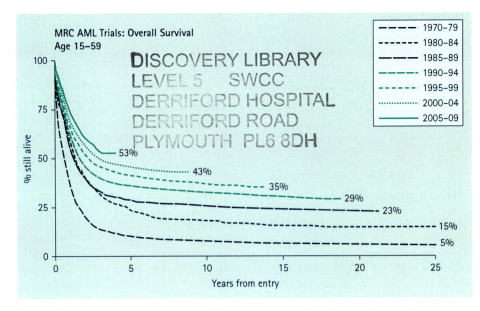

**Figure 16.1** Outcome of young adults with AML treated within Medical Research Council clinical trials from 1970–2004 (unpublished data reproduced by permission of Professor Alan Burnett).

all such patients. Recent progress has been made through improved understanding of disease biology in relation to outcome from carefully designed phase III clinical trials and has now created an increasingly refined process of disease classification[1] and risk stratification.[2,3]

Contemporary risk assessment is calculated from a combination of factors identified as strongly predictive for outcome from logistic regression multivariate analysis of large, randomized clinical trials. The paradigm for such studies are the UK Medical Research Council (MRC) AML trials, the most informative of these being AML 10/12 (younger adults and children) and AML 11/14 (older patients >60 years).

Cytogenetics is consistently the strongest predictor of clinical outcome in AML. Analysis of the MRC AML 10 trial defined three cytogenetic risk groups:

1 favourable outcome with translocations t(15;17) and t(8;21) and the inversion inv(16);
2 adverse risk with −7, −5, abnormal chromosome 3 and complex karyotype (≥5 cytogenetic abnormalities);
3 standard risk with all other patients including normal karyotype.[3]

In patients aged <60 years, the proportion of individuals in these three risk groups is 23%, 61% and 16%, respectively.[3] Overall survival at 5 years is 61%–69%, 23%–60% and 4%–21%, respectively.[3] These data have been confirmed by other study groups, although some karyotypes are categorized into different subgroups. Overall survival at 5 years in the Cancer and Leukemia Group B (CALGB) study was 55%, 24% and 5% for their favourable, intermediate and adverse karyotype groups, respectively.

Thus this patient will be classified as standard risk, based on a standard-risk karyotype. The addition of simple clinical parameters, such as response after therapy course 1, will further refine this risk stratification.[2] Preliminary data indicate that a scoring system comprising white cell count, age, sex, secondary versus *de novo* disease, cytogenetics and response after course 1 will produce a more precise stratification, principally moving approximately 15% of patients from standard to poor risk and 10% of patients from poor to standard risk.

> The patient was treated with standard induction chemotherapy consisting of two courses of (a) daunorubicin 45 mg/m² × 3 doses plus cytosine arabinoside 100 mg twice daily for 10 days followed by (b) daunorubicin 45 mg/m² × 3 doses plus cytosine arabinoside 100 mg twice daily for 8 days. Morphological remission was documented after course 1. Post-remission consolidation was two courses of high-dose cytosine arabinoside 3 g/m² twice daily for 3 days.
>
> **What is the optimal post-remission strategy in standard-risk AML?**

The options for post-remission therapy in younger patients are continuing intensive chemotherapy alone or following it by stem cell transplantation (SCT). For patients with favourable-risk AML, the potential benefits of SCT are outweighed by the risks, whilst in adverse-risk AML, SCT (allogeneic) in first complete remission (CR1) is associated with an improved outcome in recent studies, at least in younger patients (age <40 years). In standard-risk AML the optimal post-remission strategy remains unclear. An increasing body of evidence supports a role for allogeneic SCT in CR1 in younger patients (age <40 years),[4] with reduction in relapse risk outweighing the increased procedure-related mortality in comparison with chemotherapy alone, to produce an improvement in overall survival. Whether allogeneic SCT improves the poorer prognosis for patients with *FLT3* internal tandem duplication (*FLT3*-ITD; see below) remains uncertain. Ongoing international phase III studies are evaluating earlier allogeneic SCT in younger patients (age <35 years) and reduced-intensity conditioned SCT in older 'young' patients. Data from CALGB support the use of four consolidation courses of high-dose cytosine arabinoside or autografting in the post-remission setting,[5] although autografting has now fallen out of favour.

# Recent Developments

Molecular analysis of large cohorts of AML patients has revealed prognostically important acquired abnormalities of DNA and RNA. Genomic (DNA) defects comprise mutations, whilst RNA abnormalities are observed as altered gene expression either at individual gene transcriptomes or of global gene-expression patterns. Several of these abnormalities have clear prognostic significance in cytogenetically normal (CN) AML.[6]

1  *FLT3* gene mutation. Internal tandem genomic duplication or point mutations in the activation loop sequence are common, occurring in 28–33% and 5–14% of CN patients, respectively. Internal tandem duplications are of variable length but are always in-frame and produce a protein with constitutive dimerization and activation. Several studies demonstrate an adverse prognosis associated with *FLT3*-ITD in this subgroup, with similar CR rates but higher relapse rates and reduced overall survival. The prognostic significance of *FLT3* gene mutation is less clear.

2  Nucleophosmin (*NPM1*) gene mutation. Most commonly a 4–base pair duplication in exon 12, this mutation can be easily detected by gene scanning and produces a frame-shifted protein variant. The most prevalent gene mutation yet described in AML, *NPM1* mutation is found in 40%–60% of CN patients.[7] Patient characteristics include higher white blood cell count, predominance of female sex and low/absent CD34 expression. In contrast to *FLT3* mutation, *NPM1* gene mutation confers an improved prognosis in CN AML. Although overall survival is not consistently improved, CR rates are increased and event-free survival (EFS) is longer in patients with the mutation.[7]

3  *MLL* partial tandem duplication (PTD) consists of a duplication of exons 5–11 inserted into exon 4 of the *MLL* gene. This allows transcription of a functional pro-tein but is associated with epigenetic silencing of the wild-type allele. Only 8% of CN AML patients have this mutation, but most studies show a shorter CR duration but no consistent effect on CR rate, EFS or overall survival.[8]

4  *CEBPA* gene mutations may affect the C-terminus, resulting in a functional protein lacking DNA binding and homodimerization activity, or the N-terminus, encoding a non-functional protein with dominant negative activity. This class of mutations is present in 15%–19% of CN patients and confers a favourable outcome.

5  Some mutation *combinations* are mutually exclusive, for example *MLL*-PTD and *CEBPA* or *NPM1* mutation. The most common mutations, namely *FLT3*-ITD and *NPM1*, are not mutually exclusive. A favourable prognosis for *NPM1* mutation is evident in the absence of *FLT3*-ITD but it remains uncertain if *NPM1* mutation improves the poorer outcome associated with *FLT3*-ITD when the *FLT3*-ITD and *NPM1* mutation are present together.

6  The prognostic value of expression of specific genes such as *BAALC* or ETS-related gene (*ERG*) has been suggested from initial studies but needs independent

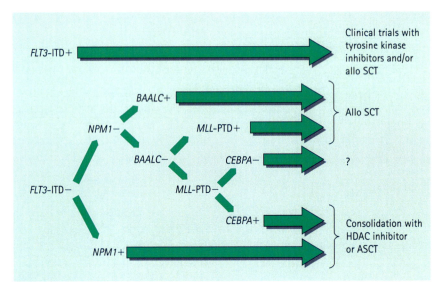

**Figure 16.2** Post-remission management strategy for CN AML. allo, allogeneic; HDAC, histone deacetylase; ASCT, autologous stem cell transplantation.[6]

validation. Similarly, although global gene-expression profiles also suggest prognostic potential in CN AML,[9] further prospective study is required.

A post-remission management strategy for CN AML is shown in Figure 16.2.

## Conclusion

Molecular and cytogenetic characterization of AML now influences clinical management. Primarily these biological characteristics determine the post-remission strategy but ongoing studies will address the influence of molecular characteristics on remission rates as well as relapse.

## Further Reading

1 Bennett JM. World Health Organization classification of the acute leukemias and myelodysplastic syndrome. *Int J Hematol* 2000; **72**: 131–3.

2 Wheatley K, Burnett AK, Goldstone AH, *et al*. A simple, robust, validated and highly predictive index for the determination of risk-directed therapy in acute myeloid leukaemia derived from the MRC AML 10 trial. United Kingdom Medical Research Council's Adult and Childhood Leukaemia Working Parties. *Br J Haematol* 1999; **107**: 69–79.

3 Grimwade D, Walker H, Oliver F, *et al*. The importance of diagnostic cytogenetics on outcome in AML: analysis of 1,612 patients entered into the MRC AML 10 trial. The Medical Research Council Adult and Children's Leukaemia Working Parties. *Blood* 1998; **92**: 2322–33.

4 Burnett AK, Wheatley K, Goldstone AH, *et al*. The value of allogeneic bone marrow transplant in patients with acute myeloid leukaemia at differing risk of relapse: results of the UK MRC AML 10 trial. *Br J Haematol* 2002; **118**: 385–400.

5 Farag SS, Ruppert AS, Mrózek K, *et al*. Outcome of induction and postremission therapy in younger adults with acute myeloid leukemia with normal karyotype: a cancer and leukemia group B study. *J Clin Oncol* 2005; **23**: 482–93.

6 Mrozek K, Marcucci G, Paschka P, Whitman SP, Bloomfield CD. Clinical relevance of mutations and gene-expression changes in adult acute myeloid leukemia with normal cytogenetics: are we ready for a prognostically prioritized molecular classification? *Blood* 2007; **109**: 431–48.

7 Falini B, Mecucci C, Tiacci E, *et al*. Cytoplasmic nucleophosmin in acute myelogenous leukemia with a normal karyotype. *N Engl J Med* 2005; **352**: 254–66.

8 Caligiuri MA, Strout MP, Lawrence D, *et al*. Rearrangement of ALL1 (MLL) in acute myeloid leukemia with normal cytogenetics. *Cancer Res* 1998; **58**: 55–9.

9 Bullinger L, Dohner K, Bair E, *et al*. Use of gene-expression profiling to identify prognostic subclasses in adult acute myeloid leukemia. *N Engl J Med* 2004; **350**: 1605–16.

**PROBLEM**

# 17  Paediatric acute lymphoblastic leukaemia

## Case History

A 14-year-old boy presented to his General Practitioner (GP) with a 2-week history of a dry cough. This was worse on exertion. He was treated with inhaled bronchodilators. The symptoms did not improve. Ten days later he returned to the GP complaining of fevers, tiredness and a skin rash. On examination he appeared pale and unwell, had a fever of 37.8°C, purpura on the feet and ankles and mild hepatosplenomegaly. He was referred to hospital. Chest X-ray revealed a widened superior mediastinum and a small right-sided pleural effusion. Full blood count was abnormal: haemoglobin 10.2 g/dl, white blood cell (WBC) count $73 \times 10^9$/l, neutrophils $0.8 \times 10^9$/l, platelets $23 \times 10^9$/l. The peripheral blood film revealed a monomorphic population of lymphoblasts and associated neutropenia and thrombocytopenia. Bone marrow aspirate confirmed the suspicion of acute lymphoblastic leukaemia (ALL) (Figure 17.1). Immunophenotyping confirmed T-cell ALL.

**What is the current approach to management of this condition?**

**What factors affect prognosis?**

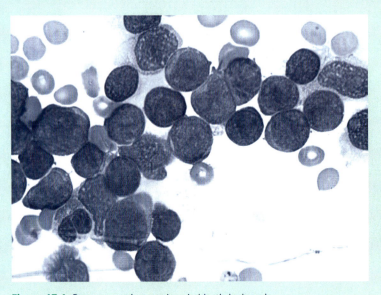

**Figure 17.1** Bone marrow in acute lymphoblastic leukaemia.

# Background

Acute lymphoblastic leukaemia is the commonest childhood malignancy, accounting for 35% of cases; 400–500 cases of ALL are diagnosed in children per year in the UK.[1] There is a peak in incidence between the ages of 2 and 5 years. Children present with bone marrow failure (anaemia, neutropenia and thrombocytopenia) due to the proliferation of abnormal lymphoid cells (blasts) in the bone marrow. T-cell immunophenotype is associated with chest disease, which may present with large mediastinal lymphadenopathy often with pleural effusion. Occasionally this may be associated with superior vena cava obstruction.

It has long been thought that there is an association between infection (as a second event) and the development of ALL in individuals with a predisposition to develop ALL, known as the Greaves hypothesis.[2] There is now molecular evidence that this is initiated *in utero*.[3,4] It is postulated that there is an abnormality/dysregulation of the immune system such that in individuals destined to develop ALL, an exposure to an otherwise innocuous infection in early childhood stimulates an extreme response in the form of immature lymphoid cells, i.e. lymphoblasts (ALL). A recent publication[5] has shown that there is an increase in the number of infections in very early childhood (including the neonatal period) in children who later develop ALL, compared with controls, suggesting an underlying abnormality of the immune system.

Immunophenotyping of lymphoblasts at diagnosis categorizes patients into ALL of B- or T-cell lineage by virtue of CD protein expression.

Good risk features include age <10 years, low WBC count at diagnosis ($<50 \times 10^9$/l), CD10 expression (common ALL antigen), t(12;21) translocation (*TEL/AML1*) molecular cytogenetic abnormality, high hyperdiploidy and rapid early response to therapy (<25% bone marrow blasts at day 15 of therapy).

Poor-risk features include age >10 years, high WBC count at diagnosis, haemoglobin >10 g/dl at diagnosis, male gender, T-lineage disease, t(9;22) (Philadelphia chromosome), near haploidy, t(4;11), intrachromosomal amplification of chromosome 21 (iAMP21) and slow early response to therapy (>25% bone marrow blasts at day 8 of therapy).

Acute lymphoblastic leukaemia in the adult population (age >18 years) is much rarer and survival much less good. Teenagers/young adults seem to constitute a different group both for current known indicators of prognosis and response to therapy, falling between the peak of presentation in children (2–5 years) and in adults (median 55 years).[6] Although there are some similarities between childhood ALL and ALL seen in older patient groups, it is difficult to understand how the same predisposition to development of ALL in relation to infection results in diagnosis at such a late stage. Either the initiating event is occurring much later or there is a different mechanism perhaps relating to different acquired cytogenetic changes. This may impact on the response to therapy.

# Recent Developments

Survival rates in childhood ALL are now >75% due to stratification of therapy based upon currently recognized markers of prognosis and response to treatment. Indeed, event-free survival (EFS) is >90% in the very best risk group. In the UK and USA, children are stratified according to age and presenting WBC count to receive standard-risk therapy (<10 years of age and WBC count <50 × 10⁹/l) or intermediate-risk therapy (>10 years and/or WBC count >50 × 10⁹/l). Slow early responders (day 15 for standard therapy and day 8 for intermediate therapy) are transferred onto a more intensive high-risk therapy regimen. Response to therapy is also monitored by assessment of minimal residual disease (MRD) by molecular methods.

Non-responders at day 28 (end of induction) have a very poor outlook.

Intensive chemotherapy regimens are associated with late effects of therapy (late side effects); this is more likely to be seen in younger children. This is particularly the case with anthracycline therapy. There is a need, therefore, to provide very long-term monitoring of late effects (cardiac function, endocrine function, bone mineral density, fertility and second malignancies).

In general, there is an increase in poor prognostic features with increasing age. The proportion of T-cell immunophenotype and presence of t(9;22) both increase with age; t(9;22) is seen in 2%–3% of childhood ALL[7] increasing to >20% in older adults. As a result, the EFS in the young and older adult populations is considerably worse than that of children under 10 years of age or in the age range 10–15 years. However, a recent analysis of a high-risk ALL trial from the USA showed that young adult patients (age 16–21 years) with high hyperdiploidy had an excellent outcome.

Several recent studies have shown that young adults with ALL have better remission rates and disease-free survival when treated on so-called 'paediatric' treatment regimens compared with those treated on 'adult' treatment regimens.[8] There are differences in the types of chemotherapy used, with a much greater emphasis on vincristine, steroids and asparaginase in 'paediatric' protocols than in 'adult' protocols. However. treatment-related morbidity (toxicity) and mortality is also greater in older patients receiving 'paediatric' protocols, especially death in induction and in first remission, steroid-induced diabetes and avascular necrosis of bone, and asparaginase-induced pancreatitis.

Thus despite the conventional risk stratification, there seems to be an overlap between age and outcome, with some poor responders in the young age group and some good responders in the older age groups. There is an implication that there is still more that we need to know to define more accurately the most appropriate therapy for specific individuals.

Bone marrow transplantation is indicated in those with adverse features: Philadelphia chromosome, near haploidy, non-responders at day 28 who subsequently achieve remission and those who relapse on treatment or within two years from end of therapy.

## Conclusion

In this case history, cytogenetic analysis of the bone marrow was normal. He was assessed as being of intermediate risk and treated with the nationally agreed children's ALL protocol. This consists of four drugs (vincristine, dexamethasone, daunorubicin and asparaginase) and intrathecal methotrexate. A bone marrow reassessment at day 28 showed that he was in remission.

Treatment continued with consolidation therapy (cyclophosphamide, cytosine and intrathecal methotrexate), interim maintenance, two courses of intensification therapy with a further course of interim maintenance therapy in between. The remaining (almost two and one-half years) was maintenance therapy with daily oral mercaptopurine, weekly oral methotrexate with monthly intravenous vincristine, and a 5-day course of dexamethasone. The patient had a human leukocyte antigen (HLA)-identical sibling and would be considered for allogeneic transplantation if he relapses within two years of completing maintenance therapy.

## Further Reading

1  Stiller CA, Eatock EM. Patterns of care and survival for children with acute lymphoblastic leukaemia diagnosed between 1980 and 1994. *Arch Dis Child* 1999; **81**: 202–8.

2  Greaves M. Infection, immune responses and the aetiology of childhood leukaemia. *Nat Rev Cancer* 2006; **6**: 193–203.

3  Greaves MF, Maia AT, Wiemels JL, Ford AM. Leukemia in twins: lessons in natural history. *Blood* 2003; **102**: 2321–33.

4  Greaves MF, Wiemels J. Origins of chromosome translocations in childhood leukemia. *Nat Rev Cancer* 2003; **3**: 639–49.

5  Roman E, Simpson J, Ansell P, *et al.* Childhood acute lymphoblastic leukemia and infections in the first year of life: a report from the United Kingdom Childhood Cancer Study. *Am J Epidemiol* 2007; **165**: 496–504.

6  Chessells JM, Hall E, Prentice HG, Durrant J, Bailey CC, Richards SM. The impact of age on outcome in lymphoblastic leukaemia: MRC UKALL X and Xa compared. *Leukemia* 1998; **12**: 463–73.

7  Jones LK, Saha V. Philadelphia positive acute lymphoblastic leukaemia of childhood. *Br J Haematol* 2005; **130**: 489–500.

8  Plasschaert SLA, Kamps WA, Vellenga E, de Vries EG, de Bont ES. Prognosis in childhood and adult acute lymphoblastic leukaemia: a question of maturation? *Cancer Treat Rev* 2004; **30**: 37–51.

# 18 Adult acute lymphoblastic leukaemia

## Case History

A 32-year-old Polish plumber with a young family is receiving treatment for Philadelphia-positive acute lymphoblastic leukaemia (Ph⁺ ALL) and has achieved complete remission (CR) with induction therapy. He has no siblings but has been offered a stem cell transplantation (SCT) if a suitable unrelated donor can be identified. He is concerned about the risk of transplant and the long-term side effects.

**What are the chances of finding a suitable donor?**

**Is he likely to benefit from a transplant?**

**What are the likely long-term complications of transplantation?**

## Background

Acute lymphoblastic leukaemia (ALL) is rare, with 730 new cases diagnosed annually in the UK. Peaks of incidence occur under the age of 5 years, during the middle thirties and at over 60 years. The appearance of an aberrant chromosome 22, the Philadelphia chromosome, resulting from a reciprocal translocation t(9;22), is the classic founding event of chronic myeloid leukaemia (CML). However, the Philadelphia chromosome is frequently found in ALL lymphoblasts, accounting for 14% of patients presenting between the ages of 25 and 35 years.[1] The translocation produces the *BCR-ABL* fusion gene that encodes a constitutively active tyrosine kinase contributing to malignant transformation in Ph⁺ ALL.

Due to high relapse rates, patients with Ph⁺ ALL fare worse than their Ph⁻ counterparts and 5-year disease-free survival (DFS) following standard chemotherapy is less than 10% compared to 30%–65% in Ph⁻ ALL.

Haemopoietic SCT permits high doses of cytotoxic therapy to be given, since the principle toxicity of such therapy – bone marrow failure – is ameliorated by infusion of stem cells shortly after high-dose therapy is completed. Autologous stem cells may be obtained from the patient prior to high-dose therapy but may be contaminated by tumour cells. Allogeneic stem cells, derived from a donor, are tumour free and may mediate a 'graft-versus-leukaemia' (GvL) effect. Genetic disparity between patient and donor influences the incidence of graft rejection, GvL and graft-versus-host disease (GvHD) that may complicate allogeneic SCT. Donor suitability is primarily dictated by the genetic constraints of the human leukocyte antigen (HLA) system. Three loci are key to selection and donors should ideally be identical to the patient at each HLA-A, HLA-B and HLA-DR pair. Siblings inherit one haplotype from each parent and have a theoretical chance of 1/4 of being a '6/6' match with one another. It is customary to type volunteer unrelated donors at several additional loci since many other alleles, likely to be mismatched in an unrelated donor, exert an influence on the potential outcomes of SCT. The chances of finding a suitable unrelated donor within the international donor registries are frequently better than 80% but are influenced by the ethnicity of the patient, as most registered donors are of Northern European origin.

Myeloablative therapy, combining total body irradiation (TBI) and chemotherapy, followed by donor SCT has been successful in eradicating Ph+ ALL, with long-term DFS of 27%–46% when performed in first complete remission. Transplant-related mortality (TRM) has fallen due to improved supportive care and donor selection but 30% of patients relapse post-SCT and prognosis is then poor.[2]

# Recent Developments

While the first hurdle to SCT donor identification is genetic variation, additional factors such as donor age, sex, parity and health are significant in terms of practical access to the donated stem cells and also the impact on post-SCT complications such as GvHD. Umbilical cord blood (UCB) stem cells that are obtained at delivery, HLA-typed and cryopreserved are readily accessible. The absolute numbers of stem cells in individual UCB donations are relatively low and in practice this limits most UCB SCT to paediatric practice, since the number of stem cells required for SCT is a function of recipient weight. However, the realization that HLA-matching requirements for cord-blood donations are less stringent than for adult donors, plus the demonstrable success of SCT in adults using pooled multiple UCB donations,[3] has increased the chances of identifying a suitable unrelated SCT donation to more than 95%.

Intense myeloablative preparative regimens can, in association with the GvL effect of allogeneic SCT, eradicate Ph+ ALL but are also responsible for late complications of SCT. The requirement for lifelong surveillance is well established in paediatric practice and recognition of its importance in adult SCT survivors is leading to the development of 'late effects clinics'. Common late effects of myeloablative regimens, especially those that incorporate TBI, are infertility (sperm banking prior to chemotherapy should be discussed), cataracts (ubiquitous, unless fractionated TBI is given) and hypothyroidism (15%). The risk of solid tumours occurring several years post-SCT is two- to threefold that of age-matched controls. Chronic GvHD may also be debilitating and life threatening. Systematic evaluation of patients in long-term remission has led to recognition of additional therapy-induced late effects such as delayed pulmonary disease, renal impairment and autoimmune disease.

The belief that toxicity of SCT may be reduced, while retaining the valuable GvL effect, has underpinned recent reductions in the intensity of preparative therapy pre-SCT without compromising engraftment. Transplant-related mortality within three months of SCT appears improved in these reduced-intensity regimens but a full analysis of such regimens will require longer follow-up and prospective clinical trials.

Imatinib, a tyrosine kinase inhibitor (TKI) that targets the constitutively active ABL kinase found in Ph+ leukaemias, has generated a seismic advance in the initial treatment of CML, with 89% 5-year overall survival (OS) achieved. Imatinib has proved beneficial too in the treatment of Ph+ ALL, and when added to standard chemotherapy increased

CR rates to 96%[4] and OS at 1 year to 66%–85%.[4,5] Maintenance therapy with imatinib may reduce relapse rates, permits some flexibility in planning of SCT for eligible patients and may improve the quality of CR at the time of SCT by reducing residual Ph+ ALL cells. Use of a combination of chemotherapy and imatinib followed by allogeneic SCT has yielded OS of 73% at 1 year[4] and relapse rates may be reduced by imatinib maintenance post-SCT. Resistance of CML cells to imatinib may be circumvented using a second-generation TKI but this is less clear in Ph+ ALL.[6] Establishing the future roles of allogeneic SCT and TKIs in the treatment of Ph+ ALL requires longer follow-up.

## Conclusion

It is highly likely that a suitable unrelated donor will be identified for this patient. Current understanding of the response of Ph+ ALL to therapy would recommend a combination of chemotherapy plus imatinib followed by a myeloablative TBI-based preparative regimen, matched unrelated donor SCT and imatinib maintenance thereafter. This is the approach of the current Medical Research Council UKALL 12 clinical trial for Ph+ ALL. However, in the future, the role of combination chemotherapy plus TKI with or without SCT, and the place of reduced-intensity SCT, may be clearer.[7] All patients with Ph+ ALL should be offered the opportunity to participate in clinical trials whenever possible.

## Further Reading

1 Secker-Walker LM, Craig JM, Hawkins JM, Hoffbrand AV. Philadelphia positive acute lymphoblastic leukemia in adults: age distribution, BCR breakpoint and prognostic significance. *Leukemia* 1991; **5**: 196–9.

2 Ottmann OG, Wassmann B. Treatment of Philadelphia chromosome-positive acute lymphoblastic leukemia. *Hematology Am Soc Hematol Educ Program* 2005; 118–22.

3 Barker JN, Weisdorf DJ, DeFor TE, *et al.* Transplantation of 2 partially HLA-matched umbilical cord blood units to enhance engraftment in adults with hematologic malignancy. *Blood* 2005; **105**: 1343–7.

4 Yanada M, Takeuchi J, Sugiura I, *et al.* High complete remission rate and promising outcome by combination of imatinib and chemotherapy for newly diagnosed BCR-ABL-positive acute lymphoblastic leukemia: a phase II study by the Japan Adult Leukemia Study Group. *J Clin Oncol* 2006; **24**: 460–66.

5 Delannoy A, Delabesse E, Lhéritier V, *et al.* Imatinib and methylprednisolone alternated with chemotherapy improve the outcome of elderly patients with Philadelphia-positive acute lymphoblastic leukemia: results of the GRAALL AFR09 study. *Leukemia* 2006; **20**: 1526–32.

6 Williams RT, Roussel MF, Sherr CJ. ARF gene loss enhances oncogenicity and limits imatinib response in mouse models of BCR-ABL-induced acute lymphoblastic leukemia. *Proc Natl Acad Sci USA* 2006; **103**: 6688–93.

7 Hahn T, Wall D, Camitta B, *et al.* The role of cytotoxic therapy with hematopoietic stem cell transplantation in the therapy of acute lymphoblastic leukemia in adults: an evidence-based review. *Biol Blood Marrow Transplant* 2006; **12**: 1–30.

# 19 Chronic lymphocytic leukaemia – early stage disease

## Case History

A 56-year-old man presented with dysuria and during the investigation had a full blood count that was abnormal. The dysuria settled spontaneously. He was otherwise well with no symptoms and no weight loss, lethargy or sweats. He had no previous medical history of note. He was on no drugs. He had two brothers who were both well and a sister who was diagnosed with chronic lymphocytic leukaemia (CLL) at the age of 52 years. Clinical examination was entirely normal with, specifically, no palpable lymph nodes, liver or spleen. At presentation his white cell count was $14.3 \times 10^9$/l, neutrophils $2.4 \times 10^9$/l, lymphocytes $8 \times 10^9$/l, haemoglobin 15.1 g/dl and platelets $339 \times 10^9$/l.

**What is the most likely cause of his lymphocytosis?**

**What investigations would you perform?**

**Could there be a link between his disease and his sister's CLL?**

**How would you manage his case?**

## Background

The differential diagnosis for this patient's lymphocytosis lies between a reactive process, which seems unlikely as he is obviously well, or a chronic lymphoproliferative disorder, such as CLL.[1] A blood film was examined which revealed a large number of small, mature lymphocytes and frequent smear cells but was otherwise normal. Immunophenotyping performed by flow cytometry on his peripheral blood revealed that the majority of his lymphocytes were monoclonal with the following immunophenotype: CD19[+], CD5[+], CD23[+], CD20[weak], CD38[+], surface immunoglobulin $\kappa^{\text{weak}}$. Therefore a diagnosis of CLL

| Stage | Organ enlargement* | Haemoglobin (g/dl)** | | Platelets ($\times 10^9$/l) |
|---|---|---|---|---|
| A | 0, 1 or 2 areas | ≥10 | AND | ≥100 |
| B | 3, 4 or 5 areas | ≥10 | AND | ≥100 |
| C | Not considered | <10 | OR | <100 |

Table 19.1 Binet staging system

*Each of the following count as one: lymph nodes >1cm in the neck, axillae or groin, palpable liver or spleen.
**Secondary causes of anaemia (i.e. iron deficiency) must be identified and treated before staging.

was established and he has early stage disease (Binet's stage A; Table 19.1).[2] The main differential diagnosis is another chronic lymphoproliferative disorder, such as mantle cell lymphoma or marginal zone lymphoma.

In CLL there is a familial risk, with approximately 3% of patients having a first-degree family member with CLL and a small number of families with several members suffering from CLL. In fact even in apparently 'normal' members (those with no clinical or blood-count evidence of CLL) of families with CLL there is a very high incidence of 'subclinical' CLL indicating a clear increase in risk.[3] Familial CLL is not directly inherited and it appears that individuals probably inherit a predisposition to develop CLL, although no specific gene has been identified to date. Several genes have been implicated as having a role in CLL in a recent publication.[4]

No therapy has been shown to provide a survival benefit if given to stage A CLL patients early rather than waiting until the disease progresses.[5]

Therefore the correct management in this case is to watch and wait.

The patient remained well in himself over the next 2 years but there was a steady and progressive increase in his lymphocyte count. After 2 years he developed generalized lymphadenopathy with lymph glands up to 5 cm in diameter, hepatosplenomegaly, a falling platelet count and anaemia. At this time his full blood count was white blood cells $153 \times 10^9/l$, lymphocytes $147 \times 10^9/l$, neutrophils $4.1 \times 10^9/l$, haemoglobin 9.7 g/dl and platelets $78 \times 10^9/l$. His direct Coombs' test (DCT) was negative and his bone marrow was heavily and diffusely replaced by CLL.

**What further tests would you perform?**

**Does he require treatment and, if so, with what therapy?**

He now needs treatment. His cytopenias are due to marrow replacement rather than being immune mediated, as his DCT is negative and his marrow is replaced by CLL.

# Recent Developments

Until recently, the standard therapy, as proven by randomized controlled trials, for patients without comorbidity was fludarabine combined with cyclophosphamide (FC).[6-8] However, the German CLL Study Group CLL8 trial has now demonstrated that the addition of rituximab, the monoclonal antibody against CD20, to FC (FCR) yields much higher rates of complete remission which translate into prolonged progression-free and overall survival compared to FC alone.[9-11] Therefore the standard therapy for patients with CLL who require treatment and are considered fit enough for more intensive therapy is the combination of FCR. The only exception is for patients with poor-risk disease as defined by fluorescent *in situ* hybridization (FISH).[8,12] This poor-risk disease is defined by loss of the short arm of chromosome 17 (or 17p-), which includes the locus of the p53 gene. Chronic lymphocytic leukaemia with *p53* deletion does not respond well to chemotherapy-based treatments as these depend on the p53 pathway for their activity. There is now mounting evidence that other types of therapy that do not utilize p53 for their activity, such as steroids or monoclonal antibodies, result in better response rates for patients with 17p-.

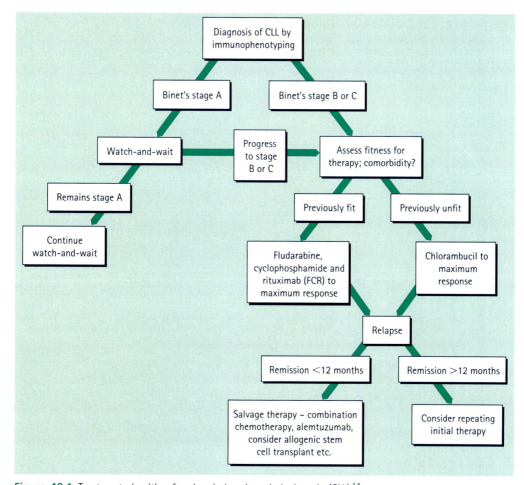

**Figure 19.1** Treatment algorithm for chronic lymphocytic leukaemia (CLL).[14]

Our patient had FISH performed, which revealed an isolated deletion of the long arm of chromosome 11 (11q-) and this abnormality was previously associated with a relatively poor risk. However, it appears that the addition of rituximab to FC in patients with 11q deletion overcomes the poor prognostic nature of this abnormality rendering these patients similar to other standard risk patients.[13] He was treated before the rituximab trial data was available and therefore received six cycles of FC, achieving a complete remission. The results of the LRF CLL4 trial recently completed in the UK indicate that the median time to progression following FC is 3 years and 7 months, with a median overall survival of just over 5 years.

# Conclusion

Two-thirds of patients with CLL present with Binet's stage A disease. Approximately one-half of these patients will progress at some time to need therapy, as our patient did. He responded well to combination chemotherapy but is still likely to progress in the future and will have a shortened survival due to his CLL. There has been massive progress in our understanding of the biology of CLL and in its treatment (Figure 19.1). Compared to historical controls, survival for patients with CLL has improved and the recent advances promise to improve the outcome for future patients, with cures becoming a reasonable aim.

# Further Reading

1 Cheson BD, Bennett JM, Grever M, *et al.* National Cancer Institute-sponsored Working Group guidelines for chronic lymphocytic leukemia: revised guidelines for diagnosis and treatment. *Blood* 1996; **87**: 4990–97.

2 Binet JL, Auquier A, Dighiero G, *et al.* A new prognostic classification of chronic lymphocytic leukemia derived from a multivariate survival analysis. *Cancer* 1981; **48**: 198–206.

3 Rawstron AC, Yuille MR, Fuller J, *et al.* Inherited predisposition to CLL is detectable as subclinical monoclonal B-lymphocyte expansion. *Blood* 2002; **100**: 2289–91.

4 Di Bernardo MC, Crowther-Swanepoel D, Broderick P, *et al.* A genome-wide association study identifies six susceptibility loci for chronic lymphocytic leukemia. *Nat Genet.* 2008; **40**: 1204–10.

5 CLL Trialists' Collaborative Group. Chemotherapeutic options in chronic lymphocytic leukemia: a meta-analysis of the randomized trials. *J Natl Cancer Inst* 1999; **91**: 861–8.

6 Eichhorst BF, Busch R, Hopfinger G, *et al.* German CLL Study Group. Fludarabine plus cyclophosphamide versus fludarabine alone in first-line therapy of younger patients with chronic lymphocytic leukemia. *Blood* 2006; **107**: 885–91.

7 Flinn IW, Neuberg DS, Grever MR, *et al.* Phase III trial of fludarabine plus cyclophosphamide compared with fludarabine for patients with previously untreated chronic lymphocytic leukemia: US Intergroup Trial E2997. *J Clin Oncol* 2007; **25**: 793–8.

8 Catovsky D, Richards S, Matutes E, *et al.* Assessment of fludarabine plus cyclophosphamide for patients with chronic lymphocytic leukaemia (the LRF CLL4 Trial): a randomised controlled trial. *Lancet* 2007; **370**: 230–39.

9 Keating MJ, O'Brien S, Albitar M, *et al.* Early results of a chemoimmunotherapy regimen of fludarabine, cyclophosphamide, and rituximab as initial therapy for chronic lymphocytic leukemia. *J Clin Oncol* 2005; **23**: 4079–88.

10 Hallek M, Fingerle-Rowson G, Fink AM, *et al.* Immunochemotherapy with Fludarabine (F), Cyclophosphamide (C), and Rituximab (R) (FCR) Versus Fludarabine and Cyclophosphamide (FC) Improves Response Rates and Progression-Free Survival (PFS) of Previously Untreated Patients (pts) with Advanced Chronic Lymphocytic Leukemia (CLL) *Blood* 2008; **112**: Abstract 325.

11 Hallek M, Fingerle-Rowson G, Fink AM, *et al.* First-Line Treatment with Fludarabine (F), Cyclophosphamide (C), and Rituximab (R) (FCR) Improves Overall Survival (OS) in Previously Untreated Patients (pts) with Advanced Chronic Lymphocytic Leukemia (CLL): Results of a Randomized Phase III Trial On Behalf of An International Group of Investigators and the German CLL Study Group. *Blood* 2009; **114**: Abstract 535.

12 Döhner H, Stilgenbauer S, Benner A, *et al.* Genomic aberrations and survival in chronic lymphocytic leukemia. *N Engl J Med* 2000; **343**: 1910–16.

13 Stilgenbauer S, Zenz T, Winkler D, *et al.* Genomic Aberrations, VH Mutation Status and Outcome after Fludarabine and Cyclophosphamide (FC) or FC Plus Rituximab (FCR) in the CLL8 Trial. *Blood* 2008; **112**: Abstract 781.

14 Oscier DG, Fegan C, Hillmen P, *et al.* Guidelines on the diagnosis and management of chronic lymphocytic leukaemia. *Br J Haematol* 2004; **125**: 294–317.

# 20 Chronic lymphocytic leukaemia – advanced stage disease

## Case History

A 55-year-old man presented in 2002 with severe tiredness, developing over a period of 4 months, associated with weight loss of 5 kg and night sweats. He had no previous medical history of note and was taking no medication. He had two brothers who were both well. On examination he looked pale and had a palpable spleen 4 cm below the left costal margin. Lymph nodes were palpable up to 2 cm in diameter in both axillae and in both sides of his neck. At presentation his white cell count was $60.0 \times 10^9$/l, neutrophils $2.4 \times 10^9$/l, lymphocytes $56 \times 10^9$/l, haemoglobin 9.8 g/dl and platelets $88 \times 10^9$/l. Immunophenotyping confirmed that the lymphocytes were clonal (CD19[+], CD5[+], CD23[+], CD20[weak], surface immunoglobulin κ[weak]). His bone marrow trephine biopsy was replaced by small lymphocytes. A computed tomography scan confirmed the presence of widespread lymphadenopathy and splenomegaly. His direct Coombs' test (DCT) was negative.

**What is the diagnosis?**

**What stage is his disease?**

**How would you manage his case?**

## Background

His presentation and immunophenotyping are typical of chronic lymphocytic leukaemia (CLL).[1] He has advanced stage disease in view of his bone marrow failure (either Binet's stage C or Rai stage IV [Table 20.1] – Binet's staging system[2] is generally used in Europe and the Rai system[3] in the USA) and he therefore requires therapy. If he had presented in 2007 he would have been treated with fludarabine plus cyclophosphamide, as this has been proven in three large, randomized trials to be superior to fludarabine alone in terms of response rates and progression-free survival.[4–6] In 2009, the addition of rituximab, the monoclonal antibody to CD20, to FC (FCR) was shown to improve response rates, progression-free survival and overall survival and has now become the standard therapy for patients with CLL who require treatment and are relatively fit.[7,8] However, in 2002 these trials were in progress and he was entered into one of them, the LRF CLL4 trial. This was a randomized trial in which he was assigned to the fludarabine monotherapy arm. In 2001 the National Institute of Clinical Excellence issued a Technology Appraisal for

| Table 20.1 Rai staging system (USA) | |
|---|---|
| Stage | Definition |
| 0 | Blood lymphocyte count $15 \times 10^9$/l or more, with 40% or more lymphocytes in marrow differential count |
| I | Stage 0 plus enlarged lymph nodes |
| II | Stage 0 plus enlarged spleen, or liver, or both; lymph nodes may or may not be enlarged |
| III | Stage 0 plus anaemia (haemoglobin less than 11g/dl); nodes may or may not be enlarged |
| IV | Stage 0 plus thrombocytopenia (platelet count $100 \times 10^9$/l); organomegaly and anaemia may or may not be present |

fludarabine[9] and recommended that it should be given orally rather than intravenously at a dose of 40 mg/m$^2$/day for 5 days every 4 weeks.

He therefore received fludarabine orally at the recommended dose but after three cycles he became increasingly short of breath. At this time he still had palpable lymph nodes all less than 2 cm in diameter and his spleen was 2 cm below the costal margin. His full blood count was as follows: white cell count $14.7 \times 10^9$/l, neutrophils $1.2 \times 10^9$/l, lymphocytes $11.2 \times 10^9$/l, haemoglobin 5.8 g/dl and platelets $68 \times 10^9$/l.

**What is the likely cause of his deterioration?**

**What investigations would you perform?**

**How would you manage his case now?**

He has clearly not responded to fludarabine but has most likely developed autoimmune haemolytic anaemia (AIHA). His DCT was strongly positive for both immunoglobulin and complement. His bilirubin was raised at 27 μmol/l as was his lactate dehydrogenase (620 IU/l) but his reticulocyte count was low at $20 \times 10^9$/l. Therefore he has AIHA secondary to fludarabine therapy but he has a relatively poor marrow compensation due to his CLL and recent therapy. Fludarabine-induced haemolytic anaemia was seen in 11% of patients receiving fludarabine monotherapy in the LRF CLL4 trial, which was a similar incidence to that in the chlorambucil arm of the trial (12% of patients) but significantly higher than following fludarabine plus cyclophosphamide (5%).[6] However, AIHA secondary to fludarabine monotherapy has a tendency to be more severe, and in fact four patients in the fludarabine arm of the LRF CLL4 trial died from haemolysis compared to none in the chlorambucil or fludarabine plus cyclophosphamide arms.[10] Therefore fludarabine-induced haemolytic anaemia is a medical emergency.

He was treated with transfusions (despite cross-matching being almost impossible due to his strongly positive DCT) given by the clinical trial and prednisolone at 1 mg/kg/day. He required twelve units of red cells over the next 2 weeks but fortunately responded to the prednisolone and had the prednisolone dose reduced after 4 weeks of therapy. Eight weeks after starting his prednisolone he was taking 30 mg/day and was transfusion independent with the following blood count: white cells 27.4 × 10⁹/l, neutrophils 1.9 × 10⁹/l, lymphocytes 23.1 × 10⁹/l, haemoglobin 9.8 g/dl and platelets 79 × 10⁹/l. A bone marrow biopsy was repeated, which showed heavy involvement with CLL. Fluorescent *in situ* hydridization was performed for detection of chromosomal abnormalities and 70% of his CLL cells had a loss of the short arm of chromosome 17 (17p deletion).[11,12]

**What is the most appropriate treatment to consider?**

**What further tests would you perform?**

# Recent Developments

Patients developing fludarabine-associated haemolysis should not be re-exposed to fludarabine. In addition, the discovery of deletion of the short arm of chromosome 17 is a very poor-risk feature. This implies the loss of the *p53* oncogene, as this deletion removes one *p53* locus and, in many cases, sequencing of the remaining *p53* gene reveals a mutation. Therefore his disease will be *p53* dysfunctional. This explains why he was resistant to fludarabine, as conventional chemotherapy that depends on DNA damage or repair mechanisms, such as alkylating agents or purine analogues, requires functional *p53* to be effective. In the LRF CLL4 trial, patients with over 20% 17p- cells had a poor response rate and all had died within 4 years of starting therapy for CLL.[6]

We therefore need to consider therapies that do not depend on the *p53* pathway for their activity. These include monoclonal antibodies and high-dose steroids such as the combination of alemtuzumab and high-dose methyl prednisolone (CamPred) which has demonstrated high response rates in *p53*-deleted (17p-) CLL.[13] In addition, there are a number of other possible therapies in clinical trials at present which may be effective in *p53*-deleted CLL. The other therapy that should be considered is allogeneic stem cell transplantation (alloSCT) as our patient's prognosis is poor and alloSCT is the only therapy with curative potential in CLL. It also appears that the efficacy of alloSCT is mainly through graft-versus-CLL and this appears to be *p53* independent.[14] Therefore the patient and his brothers were tissue typed and one of his brothers was human leukocyte antigen (HLA)-matched with the patient.

The patient was treated with alemtuzumab, which is a monoclonal antibody targeting the CD52 antigen, which has been shown to be effective for fludarabine-refractory CLL. In addition, there is good evidence that the response rates in 17p deleted CLL are the same as for non-17p deleted cases and we would expect high response rates for patients with relatively non-bulky lymphadenopathy, such as our patient. He responded well after 12 weeks of intravenous alemtuzumab and achieved a complete remission, although he had a low level of CLL detectable in his bone marrow by four-colour flow cytometry for minimal residual disease (MRD). After an interval of 3 months he underwent a reduced-intensity allogeneic stem cell transplant from his HLA-matched brother. He engrafted at day +16 post-transplant and at his day 100 assessment had no detectable residual disease by flow cytometry (MRD negative). He remains well 2 years post-transplant.

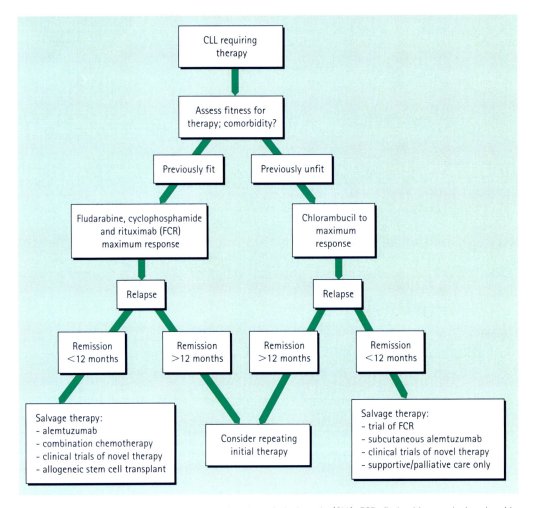

**Figure 20.1** Treatment algorithm for chronic lymphocytic leukaemia (CLL). FCR, fludarabine, cyclophosphamide and rituximab.

## Conclusion

The patient presented with advanced CLL requiring therapy (Figure 20.1) and received fludarabine monotherapy within a randomized phase III clinical trial. He developed severe autoimmune haemolysis secondary to fludarabine, which fortunately responded to therapy. However, he had biologically poor-risk CLL (loss of the *p53* gene from his leukaemia cells) and required therapy targeted to avoid dependence on the *p53* pathway, in this case alemtuzumab. He subsequently successfully underwent an allogeneic stem cell transplantation, which is a therapy used only in a small minority of patients with CLL but should be considered in selected patients, particularly those with biologically poor-risk disease.

# Further Reading

1  Oscier DG, Fegan C, Hillmen P, *et al.* Guidelines on the diagnosis and management of chronic lymphocytic leukaemia. *Br J Haematol* 2004; **125**: 294–317.

2  Binet JL, Auquier A, Dighiero G, *et al.* A new prognostic classification of chronic lymphocytic leukemia derived from a multivariate survival analysis. *Cancer* 1981; **48**: 198–206.

3  Rai KR, Sawitsky A, Cronkite EP, Chanana AD, Levy RN, Pasternack BS. Clinical staging of chronic lymphocytic leukemia. *Blood* 1975; **46**: 219–34.

4  Eichhorst BF, Busch R, Hopfinger G, *et al.* German CLL Study Group. Fludarabine plus cyclophosphamide versus fludarabine alone in first-line therapy of younger patients with chronic lymphocytic leukemia. *Blood* 2006; **107**: 885–91.

5  Flinn IW, Neuberg DS, Grever MR, *et al.* Phase III trial of fludarabine plus cyclophosphamide compared with fludarabine for patients with previously untreated chronic lymphocytic leukemia: US Intergroup Trial E2997. *J Clin Oncol* 2007; **25**: 793–8.

6  Catovsky D, Richards S, Matutes E, *et al.* Assessment of fludarabine plus cyclophosphamide for patients with chronic lymphocytic leukaemia (the LRF CLL4 Trial): a randomised controlled trial. *Lancet* 2007; **370**: 230–39.

7  Hallek M, Fingerle-Rowson G, Fink AM, *et al.* Immunochemotherapy with Fludarabine (F), Cyclophosphamide (C), and Rituximab (R) (FCR) Versus Fludarabine and Cyclophosphamide (FC) Improves Response Rates and Progression-Free Survival (PFS) of Previously Untreated Patients (pts) with Advanced Chronic Lymphocytic Leukemia (CLL) *Blood* 2008; **112**: Abstract 325.

8  Hallek M, Fingerle-Rowson G, Fink AM, *et al.* First-Line Treatment with Fludarabine (F), Cyclophosphamide (C), and Rituximab (R) (FCR) Improves Overall Survival (OS) in Previously Untreated Patients (pts) with Advanced Chronic Lymphocytic Leukemia (CLL): Results of a Randomized Phase III Trial On Behalf of An International Group of Investigators and the German CLL Study Group. *Blood* 2009; **114**: Abstract 535.

9  National Institute for Clinical Excellence. Fludarabine for the treatment of B-cell chronic lymphocytic leukaemia. NICE Technology Appraisal TA29, 2001. www.nice.org.uk/guidance/

10  Dearden C, Wade R, Else M, *et al.* The prognostic significance of a positive direct antiglobulin test in chronic lymphocytic leukemia: a beneficial effect of the combination of fludarabine and cyclophosphamide on the incidence of hemolytic anemia. *Blood* 2008; **111**: 1820–6.

11  Döhner H, Stilgenbauer S, Benner A, *et al.* Genomic aberrations and survival in chronic lymphocytic leukemia. *N Engl J Med* 2000; **343**: 1910–16.

12  Oscier DG, Wade R, Orchard J, *et al.* Prognostic factors in the UK LRF CLL4 Trial. *Blood* 2006; **108**: Abstract 299.

13  Pettit AR, Matutes E, Dearden C, *et al.* Results of the Phase II NCRI CLL206 Trial of alemtuzumab in combination with high-dose methylprednisolone for high-risk (17p-) CLL. *Haematologica* 2009; **94**: Abstract 351.

14  Dreger P, Brand R, Milligan D, *et al.* Reduced-intensity conditioning lowers treatment-related mortality of allogeneic stem cell transplantation for chronic lymphocytic leukemia: a population-matched analysis. *Leukemia* 2005; **19**: 1029–33.

# 21 Chronic myeloid leukaemia

## Case History

A 24-year-old male presents with priapism and is found to have a grossly elevated white cell count of $450 \times 10^9/l$. Haemoglobin is 10.4 g/dl and platelets $620 \times 10^9/l$. Clinical examination reveals splenomegaly at 7 cm below the costal margin and subsequently a diagnosis of chronic myeloid leukaemia (CML) is made following bone marrow examination and cytogenetic analysis. The patient has two brothers who are fit and well.

**What would be the optimum initial management of this patient?**

**How should his response to treatment be monitored?**

**What is the role of allogeneic stem cell transplantation in the management of this condition?**

## Background

Management of CML has been revolutionized in the last few years by the emergence of tyrosine kinase inhibitors, notably imatinib mesylate, which has been shown to be superior in terms of haematological, cytogenetic and molecular responses to the previous best non-transplant treatment with interferon-$\alpha$.[1] This major advance in the management of the disease was recognized in the UK by the National Institute for Clinical Excellence in 2002, when it announced that imatinib therapy was the recommended first-line treatment for all newly diagnosed patients.[2] Subsequent follow-up of patients treated with imatinib has confirmed that cytogenetic responses are durable, with 85% of patients expected to achieve a major cytogenetic response within 1 year of therapy. Recent data that have emerged following the 5-year analysis of imatinib-treated patients have confirmed that responses are not only durable but that cytogenetic and molecular responses, as measured by reduction in quantitative real-time reverse transcription–polymerase chain reaction (RT–PCR) testing for the *BCR-ABL* gene, may improve with time.[3] The question for the management of young patients with the disease is what, if any, is the continued role for allogeneic stem cell transplantation (alloSCT).

Allogeneic stem cell transplantation is by convention the only proven curative treatment for the disease, with 5-year survival rates of 75% for sibling transplants performed in the first chronic phase of the disease within 1 year of diagnosis. However, the toxicity associated with transplantation may be increased when using an unrelated donor, and quality of life may be significantly affected by the complications of bone marrow transplantation, notably graft-versus-host disease. There are a variety of donor and transplant

| Table 21.1 The European Blood and Marrow Transplantation (EBMT) score | | |
| --- | --- | --- |
| **Risk factor** | | Score |
| **Disease stage** | chronic phase | 0 |
| | accelerated phase | 1 |
| | blast crisis | 2 |
| **Age** | <20 years | 0 |
| | 20–40 years | 1 |
| | >40 years | 2 |
| **Donor/recipient sex combination** | all others | 0 |
| | female to male | 1 |
| **Histocompatibility** | HLA-identical sibling | 0 |
| | unrelated donor | 1 |
| **Time from diagnosis to transplant** | <12 months | 0 |
| | >12 months | 1 |

factors that may impact on outcome which have been evaluated to produce a prognostic scoring system – the European Blood and Marrow Transplantation (EBMT) or 'Gratwohl' score – which may help in selecting patients for transplant based on expected outcome (Table 21.1).

There is also a disease-based prognostic scoring system for CML – the Sokal score – based on easily measured parameters such as spleen size, white cell count, basophilia and platelet count, which historically correlated with outcome in the pre-imatinib era and has been shown (as has its more refined successor, the Hasford or 'Euro' score) to also separate different groups in terms of response to imatinib. Employing these two scores may have a role in determining the appropriateness or otherwise of early allogeneic transplantation in some patients. However, a note of caution should be introduced here in that the 'adverse' effect of a high Sokal score is negated if the patient subsequently achieves a complete cytogenetic response (CCyR) on imatinib, which may justify a trial of drug therapy first in all cases. If a decision not to proceed to transplantation is made, one would want to be able to monitor closely the patients' responses so that prompt transplantation could be offered to those patients who are deemed to be 'failing' therapy.

# Recent Developments

1   The monitoring of imatinib-treated patients within the IRIS study has now established various milestones that need to be achieved for the patient to be considered as having a satisfactory response. The evidence indicates that patients achieving a CCyR have an excellent long-term survival no matter how long it takes to achieve that cytogenetic response. Looking at the rate at which a cytogenetic response is obtained would appear to predict which patients are most likely to achieve a CCyR. The earliest time at which these data are interpretable is after 6 months of therapy;

patients who have not achieved any or only a minimal (<5% Philadelphia chromosome-negative cells) cytogenetic response have only a 15% chance of achieving a CCyR by 12 months.

2   Development of techniques to accurately measure residual disease by a quantitative 'real-time' RT–PCR method has allowed the introduction of the monitoring of low levels of *BCR-ABL*, the oncogene responsible for the abnormal tyrosine kinase actively associated with CML. Recent work has shown that failure to achieve a three-log reduction in *BCR-ABL1* after 12 months of imatinib therapy, as measured in this way, predicts for a slightly increased risk of subsequent progression of the disease. These observations have been reviewed by the European Leukaemia Network, who came up with proposals for the definition of adequate responses to imatinib (Table 21.2).[4]

3   Recently there has been the emergence of new tyrosine kinase inhibitors, notably nilotinib and dasatinib. These are thought to produce responses even in patients who are resistant to imatinib due to mutations affecting ABL kinase. In the case of nilotinib this is thought to be due to the fact that structural differences, as compared with imatinib, mean that it fits less well into the ATP-binding pocket (the site of action of imatinib) and nilotinib is therefore less likely to be affected by mutations that affect the configuration of this site. These emerging options for therapy in patients not responding to imatinib may have some bearing on the decision to proceed to transplantation even if the response to 'first-line therapy' is inadequate.

**Table 21.2** European Leukaemia Network (LeukaemiaNet) guidelines (with permission)[4]

| Time | Failure | Suboptimal response | Warnings |
|---|---|---|---|
| Diagnosis | NA | NA | High risk, del9q+, ACAs in Ph+ cells |
| 3 mo after diagnosis | No HR (stable disease or disease progression) | Less than CHR | NA |
| 6 mo after diagnosis | Less than CHR, no CyR (Ph+ >95%) | Less than PCyR (Ph+ >35%) | NA |
| 12 mo after diagnosis | Less than PCyR (Ph+ >35%) | Less than CCyR | Less than MmolR |
| 18 mo after diagnosis | Less than CCyR | Less than MMolR | NA |
| Anytime | Loss of CHR*, loss of CCyR†, mutation† | ACA in Ph+ cells§, loss of ¶ MMolR§, mutation | Any rise in transcript level; other chromosome abnormalities in Ph− cells |

* To be confirmed on two occasions unless associated with progression to accelerated phase (AP)/blast crisis (BC); † to be confirmed on two occasions, unless associated with CHR loss or progression to AP/BC; * high level of insensitivity to imatinib; § to be confirmed on two occasions, unless associated with CHR or CCyR loss; ¶ low level of insensitivity to imatinib.
ACAs, additional chromosome abnormalities; CCyR, complete cytogenetic response; CHR, complete haematologic response; CyR, cytogenetic response; HR, haematologic response; MmolR, major molecular response; NA, not applicable; mo, months; PCyR, partial cytogenetic response.

## Conclusion

The excellent cytogenetic and molecular response rates to imatinib have led to the emergence of a consensus opinion that most patients should be given a trial of therapy, with early reconsideration of the transplant option should response be less than adequate.

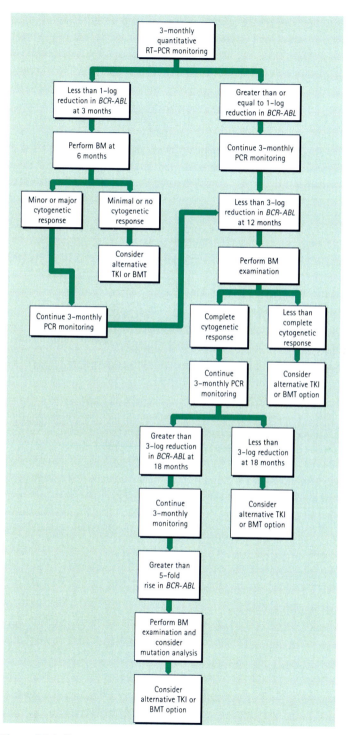

**Figure 21.1** Chronic myeloid leukaemia monitoring algorithm. BM, bone marrow; BMT, bone marrow transplant; TKI, tyrosine kinase inhibitor.

However, all patients should be assessed for suitability of early transplantation. Employing the EBMT score and Sokal score would suggest that this approach is most appropriate for those with poor disease prognostic criteria (high Sokal score) and good predicted transplant outcomes (low EBMT score). This would apply in this young man's case if either of his brothers proved to be a human leukocyte antigen (HLA) match. For all other patients, frequent monitoring of response with cytogenetics and ideally 3-monthly quantitative RT–PCR should be employed, with reconsideration of allogeneic transplantation in all those not achieving a satisfactory response. There is no evidence that imatinib is associated with an impaired post-transplant outcome although it is unclear at this stage whether delaying the transplant for greater than 1 year from diagnosis, which has been shown in previous studies to be an adverse risk factor for transplant outcome, might impact on survival. This approach to monitoring CML is summarized in Figure 21.1.

## Further Reading

1 Druker BJ, Guilhot F, O'Brien SG, *et al.* Five-year follow-up of patients receiving imatinib for chronic myeloid leukemia. *N Engl J Med* 2006; **355**: 2408–2417.

2 National Institute for Clinical Excellence. Leukaemia (chronic myloid) – imatinib. NICE Technology Appraisal TA70, 2003. www.nice.org.uk/guidance/

3 Hughes TP, Kaeda J, Branford S, *et al.* Frequency of major molecular responses to imatinib or interferon alfa plus cytarabine in newly diagnosed chronic myeloid leukemia. *N Engl J Med* 2003; **349**: 1423–32.

4 Baccarani M, Saglio G, Goldman J, *et al.* Evolving concepts in the management of chronic myeloid leukemia: recommendations from an expert panel on behalf of the European LeukemiaNet. *Blood* 2006; **108**: 1809–20.

# 22  Low-risk myelodysplastic syndrome

## Case History

A 70-year-old otherwise fit and healthy female had been diagnosed 3 years previously with myelodysplastic syndrome (MDS; French–American–British [FAB] classification subtype refractory anaemia). Cytogenetic analysis was not done, as it was considered unnecessary in this age group. The patient had a haemoglobin concentration of 7.5 g/dl, white cell count $4 \times 10^9/l$, neutrophils $2.4 \times 10^9/l$ and platelets $450 \times 10^9/l$ at diagnosis. Red cell-transfusion therapy was commenced, with a transfusion interval of 3 weekly, to temporarily relieve symptoms of anaemia. A trial of recombinant human erythropoietin therapy with 30 000 units per week for 6 weeks, escalating to 60 000 units per week for 6 weeks, produced no erythroid response. Serum ferritin assayed after 3 years of red cell-transfusion dependence was 4500 µg/l. A bone marrow examination was repeated to confirm disease stability with a view to commencing iron-chelation therapy. Serum erythropoietin concentration was 2000 IU/l. The morphology confirmed World Health Organization (WHO) classification subtype refractory cytopenia with multilineage dysplasia, which was changed to a diagnosis of 5q- syndrome when cytogenetic analysis revealed all 20 metaphases showing del(5)(q13-33) as the sole abnormality.

**Should a trial of recombinant erythropoietin have been offered?**

**Is there a therapeutic option to modify disease and promote erythropoiesis?**

## Background

The 5q- syndrome, first described by Van den Berghe in 1974 and now recognized within the WHO classification[1] as a separate nosological subtype of MDS, typically occurs in older female patients. The 5q- syndrome is a rare subtype of MDS comprising 2% of cases. However, MDS patients with the del(5q) cytogenetic abnormality and other WHO subtypes of MDS comprise a further 8% of all MDS patients.

Severe anaemia with a low/normal white cell count and a high platelet count is the typical presenting blood count profile. Bone marrow morphology is variable but characteristic monolobular megakaryocytes, relative erythroid hypoplasia and increased fibrosis are most commonly observed.[2] Karyotype analysis reveals deletion of a critical region at 5q3.1. In the 5q- syndrome this is the sole karyotypic abnormality although additional abnormalities are often seen and these confer a poorer prognosis.[2]

The prognosis is relatively good for untreated patients with 5q- syndrome, with a median survival of 10 years and a low transformation rate to acute myeloid leukaemia of 10% in 10 years. Prognosis is poorer for patients with additional karyotypic abnormalities and particularly for patients with >5% blasts in the bone marrow.

## Recent Developments

Several erythropoiesis-stimulating protein (ESP) products are now available, including the longer-acting darbepoetin alfa. No ESP is licensed for therapy in MDS. Nevertheless, worldwide it has become standard management to consider selected MDS patients for ESP therapy, based upon data from a meta-analysis of phase II trials,[3] phase II studies validating models to predict response[4] and a single small phase III trial.[5] All national guidelines for the management of MDS have recommended this therapy. Patients should be selected based upon a relatively low baseline endogenous serum erythropoietin (EPO) concentration (usually <500 IU/L) and low (two units or fewer per month) or absent red cell-transfusion requirement. Such patients have a 61% response rate to ESP.[4] Conversely, patients with serum EPO >500 IU/l and a higher red cell-transfusion requirement have a predicted response rate of 7%.

Although responses to ESP are reported in patients with 5q- syndrome, these are infrequent and most likely due to the erythroid hypoplasia and consequently very high concentrations of endogenous EPO in the majority of cases. Occasional responses to low-dose cytarabine have previously been noted. A promising new development is the high erythroid response rates reported with use of the novel immunomodulatory agent, lenalidomide, in patients with 5q- karyotypic abnormali-

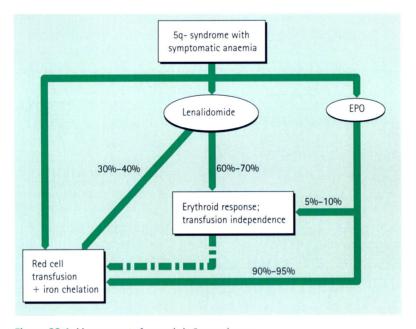

**Figure 22.1** Management of anaemia in 5q- syndrome.

ties. In a recent phase II study, 10/12 (83%) low-risk MDS patients with del(5q) achieved erythroid responses.[6] Erythroid response in a larger phase II study of similar patients is 66%.[7] Most responders achieve transfusion independence with elimination or reduction in the del(5q) clone. The median response duration is 2.2 years. Lenalidomide is myelosuppressive in the majority of cases, though other side effects occur in <10% of patients. The approach to management of anaemia in this condition is summarized in Figure 22.1.

### How should the iron overload be managed in this patient?

Strong evidence that iron overload is detrimental to outcome is lacking for patients with MDS. However, overall survival was reduced in iron-loaded patients with low-risk MDS in a recent large, retrospective cohort study.[8] For each increment in serum ferritin concentration of 500 µg/l above 1000 µg/l, overall survival was reduced by 38%. Patients dependent on transfusion since diagnosis also had poorer overall survival compared with non-transfusion-dependent patients. Although death from cardiac failure was more frequent in transfused patients, the authors do not comment on any relationship between cardiac failure and biochemical iron overload. Extrapolation from the thalassaemia literature would support a strategy of iron chelation for red cell transfusion-dependent MDS patients with a reasonably long life expectancy (>4 years), primarily patients in the Low or Intermediate-1 (Int-1) risk categories of the International Prognostic Scoring System (IPSS) and with WHO subtypes refractory anaemia (RA), refractory anaemia with ringed sideroblasts (RARS) or 5q- syndrome. The choice of iron-chelating agent remains unclear. Desferrioxamine has a safety and efficacy history spanning three decades but is cumbersome to administer by subcutaneous infusion. Deferiprone is increasingly used but side effects include gastrointestinal disturbance, erosive arthritis, neutropenia and, rarely, agranulocytosis (0.5%). Deferiprone is not licensed for MDS. Most recently licensed is a second oral agent, deferasirox, which is administered once daily and is of comparable efficacy to desferrioxamine in one phase III trial. Uncertainty about long-term side effects and high cost are legitimate obstacles to its widespread introduction into clinical practice. Of course in patients with complete erythroid response to lenalidomide, venesection is the most appropriate 'de-iron' strategy.

# Conclusion

1 All patients suspected of having a diagnosis of MDS should have karyotypic analysis, given that a targeted therapeutic option is now available.
2 Recombinant erythropoietin therapy should be considered only in patients with a high predictive response score.
3 Iron-chelation therapy should be offered to red cell transfusion-dependent MDS patients with low-risk disease and a life expectancy of at least 4 years.
4 Lenalidomide therapy should be considered for all new patients with Low/Int-1 category MDS and del(5q). Side effects, particularly myelosuppression, are significant and potentially life threatening but erythroid response is complete and durable in most patients.

# Further Reading

1 Bennett JM. World Health Organization classification of the acute leukemias and myelodysplastic syndrome. *Int J Hematol* 2000; **72**: 131–3.

2 Giagounidis AA, Germing U, Haase S, *et al.* Clinical, morphological, cytogenetic, and prognostic features of patients with myelodysplastic syndromes and del(5q) including band q31. *Leukemia* 2004; **18**: 113–9.

3 Hellström-Lindberg E. Efficacy of erythropoietin in the myelodysplastic syndromes: a meta-analysis of 205 patients from 17 studies. *Br J Haematol* 1995; **89**: 67–71.

4 Hellström-Lindberg E, Gulbrandsen N, Lindberg G, *et al.* A validated decision model for treating the anaemia of myelodysplastic syndromes with erythropoietin + granulocyte colony-stimulating factor: significant effects on quality of life. *Br J Haematol* 2003; **120**: 1037–46.

5 Casadevall N, Durieux P, Dubois S, *et al.* Health, economic, and quality-of-life effects of erythropoietin and granulocyte colony-stimulating factor for the treatment of myelodysplastic syndromes: a randomized, controlled trial. *Blood* 2004; **104**: 321–7.

6 List A, Kurtin S, Roe DJ, *et al.* Efficacy of lenalidomide in myelodysplastic syndromes. *N Engl J Med* 2005; **352**: 549–57.

7 List A, Dewald G, Bennett J, *et al.* Lenalidomide in the myelodysplastic syndrome with chromosome 5q deletion. *N Engl J Med* 2006; **355**: 1456–65.

8 Malcovati L, Porta MG, Pascutto C, *et al.* Prognostic factors and life expectancy in myelodysplastic syndromes classified according to WHO criteria: a basis for clinical decision making. *J Clin Oncol* 2005; **23**: 7594–603.

# Myeloproliferative Disorders

PROBLEM

## 23  Primary polycythaemia

## Case History

A 66-year-old woman with known mild hypertension treated with bendroflumethiazide experienced a transient ischaemic attack affecting her speech which resolved completely after about 3 hours. She had noticed occasional blurring of her vision over the past 3 months. She had not smoked for 35 years and drank eight units of alcohol weekly. Her General Practitioner commenced her on aspirin 75 mg daily. Renal and hepatic function were normal, but a blood count showed a raised haemoglobin and reduced serum erythropoietin (EPO) level (Table 23.1). The Janus kinase 2 (*JAK2*) gene was shown to be mutated.

**What is the most likely diagnosis?**

**How should the blood count abnormalities be investigated?**

**How should her condition be managed?**

## Background

The three classical chronic myeloproliferative disorders (excluding Philadelphia-positive chronic myeloid leukaemia) – polycythaemia vera (PV), idiopathic myelofibrosis (IMF) and essential thrombocythaemia (ET) – are clonal disorders with an initiating event in a pluripotent stem cell. A small proportion will transform to an acute myeloid leukaemia.

**Table 23.1 Summary of patient's investigation results**

| Parameter | Value | Units | Reference range |
| --- | --- | --- | --- |
| Haemoglobin | 19.4 | g/dl | 11.5–16.0 |
| White cell count | 7.32 | $10^9$/l | 4.0–11.0 |
| Platelets | 765 | $10^9$/l | 150–400 |
| Packed cell volume | 0.60 | | 0.37–0.47 |
| Red cell count | 7.76 | $10^{12}$/l | 3.80–5.80 |
| Mean cell volume | 74 | fl | 78–100 |
| Mean corpuscular haemoglobin | 25.0 | pg | 27.0–32.0 |
| Neutrophil count | 4.52 | $10^9$/l | 2.00–7.50 |
| Lymphocyte count | 1.33 | $10^9$/l | 1.00–4.50 |
| Monocyte count | 0.43 | $10^9$/l | 0.20–0.80 |
| Eosinophil count | 0.50 | $10^9$/l | 0.04–0.40 |
| Basophil count | 0.30 | $10^9$/l | <0.10 |
| Serum erythropoietin | 1.0 | mIU/ml | 3.0–18.0 |
| AK2 | Mutated | | |

Polycythaemia vera presents most commonly with vascular events of all types, as an incidental finding on routine blood counts and occasionally as gout. A special case of vascular event is the Budd–Chiari syndrome. Historically, the diagnosis depended on a 'points' system of major and minor criteria.[1] The major criteria were demonstration of a raised red cell volume (to distinguish true from apparent erythrocytosis), absence of a secondary cause, palpable splenomegaly and a clonality marker, e.g. cytogenetic abnormalities in the marrow. The minor criteria were neutrophilia, thrombocytosis, radiological splenomegaly, demonstration of EPO-independent erythroid colony growth and a low EPO level. Typical bone marrow morphology is shown in Figure 23.1. Polycythaemia vera has a median age of onset of 60 years with no gender distinction. The outlook for untreated PV is dismal, with a median survival of 18–24 months, the majority of deaths being due to vaso-occlusive events. The aim of treatment is to prevent vascular events and minimize transformations to acute leukaemia, a terminal event which has clearly been shown to be increased by alkylating agents and radioactive phosphorus treatment. Polycythaemia vera may also transform to myelofibrosis.

# Recent Developments

The diagnosis of the chronic myeloproliferative disorders, and PV in particular, was revolutionized in 2005 when four separate research groups identified a somatic point mutation in the *JAK2* gene which was closely associated with the chronic myeloproliferative disorders, particularly PV.[2,3] This *JAK2*$^{V617F}$ mutation represents a guanine to thymine (G→T) substitution at nucleotide 1849 in exon 14 of the gene. It occurs within the

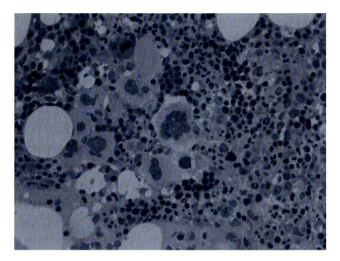

**Figure 23.1** Marrow trephine biopsy showing increased cellularity, erythroid hyperplasia and highly atypical clustered megakaryocytes typical of polycythaemia vera.

pseudokinase domain (JH2) and results in the substitution of valine to phenylalanine at codon 617. Patients, almost exclusively with PV, may show homozygosity for the mutant allele due to mitotic recombination. The $JAK2^{V617F}$ mutation causes constitutive activation of $JAK2$, and leads, via the JAK-STAT signalling pathway, to inappropriate EPO hypersensitivity or EPO-independent erythrocyte production; this aberrant pattern is more marked in patients showing homozygous mutation. Many but not all patients with PV have a low serum EPO level. $JAK2$ binds to many cytokine receptors including the thrombopoietin receptor (MPL) and the granulocyte colony-stimulating factor receptor. It is not clear why the same $JAK2^{V617F}$ mutation is implicated in the diverse clinical phenotypes of PV, ET and IMF. There is some evidence that $JAK2^{V617F}$-positive ET cases have higher haemoglobin and lower serum EPO levels than $JAK2^{V617F}$-negative cases; i.e. they resemble PV more than $JAK2^{V617F}$-negative cases.

Although the $JAK2^{V617F}$ mutation is clearly crucial in determining the general phenotype of the myeloproliferative disorders, there are several lines of evidence suggesting that the $JAK2^{V617F}$ mutation is not the primary genetic event in their causation. First, in the short time since the discovery of $JAK2^{V617F}$ it has become clear that terminal acute myeloid leukaemia is commonly V617F wild type. Secondly, careful analysis has shown that in some cases of PV there are fewer cells with the $JAK2^{V617F}$ mutation than there are with other clonal markers. Thirdly, analysis of familial myeloproliferative disorders suggests a prior initiating event.

The $JAK2^{V617F}$ mutation is detectable in the blood or marrow of 40%–60% of patients with Budd–Chiari syndrome, most of whom do not have blood count or marrow findings typical of a myeloproliferative disorder, but some of whom later develop more typical findings.[4] Using optimal testing (usually allele-specific polymerase chain reaction on DNA), at least 95% of patients with PV defined by previous criteria show the $JAK2^{V617F}$ mutation in peripheral blood neutrophil or whole blood DNA. Approximately half of the patients with ET or chronic IMF exhibit the $JAK2^{V617F}$ mutation. Currently patients with a sustained erythrocytosis should be tested for the mutation and have a serum EPO measured. The association of PV and the *JAK2*[V617F] mutation is so strong that the British guidelines for diagnosing PV have been updated specifically to take account of this.[5] A raised EPO level excludes PV except where there is a Budd–Chiari syndrome[4] or iron-deficiency anaemia with marked erythrocytosis. The causes of non-PV erythrocytosis are many and varied, requiring systematic assessment and investigation.[1]

## Management

The patient clearly has PV. The first aim of treatment is to reduce the haematocrit to within the normal range for age and gender, and this is most speedily achieved by thera-peutic venesection. Her thrombocytosis can contribute to vascular events and daily aspirin should be prescribed. Since venesection does not reduce platelets or neutrophils, long-term treatment should also include myelosuppressive therapy, especially as her age increases her risk of a thrombotic event. Hydroxycarbamide (hydroxyurea, HU) is the most commonly used myelosuppressive in the UK. It appears to have little leukae-mogenic potential and overdosage is readily reversible. Interferon alfa is also active in PV, but its use is limited by side effects. It should be considered if the patient is intolerant of HU. The patient's long-term management will involve varying use of venesection and myelosuppression tailored to her blood counts.

# Conclusion

This patient should expect a median survival approaching 20 years, a dramatic improve-ment compared to the natural history of the illness. The diagnosis of PV by detection of the *JAK2*[V617F] mutation in patients with only borderline blood count changes will further 'improve' survival. The discovery of the importance of the V617F mutation in the *JAK2* gene has revolutionized our understanding of PV and has led to a simple diagnostic test, but will pose new problems in deciding appropriate therapy in this group of patients.

# Further Reading

1   McMullin MF, Bareford D, Campbell P, *et al*. General Haematology Task Force of the British Committee for Standards in Haematology. Guidelines for the diagnosis, investigation and management of polycythaemia/erythrocytosis. *Br J Haematol* 2005; **130**: 174–95.

2   Campbell PJ, Green AR. The myeloproliferative disorders. *N Engl J Med* 2006; **355**: 2452–66.

3   Tefferi A. The diagnosis of polycythemia vera: new tests and old dictums. *Best Pract Res Clin Haematol* 2006; **19**: 455–69.

4   Patel RK, Lea NC, Heneghan MA, *et al*. Prevalence of the activating JAK2 tyrosine kinase mutation V617F in the Budd–Chiari syndrome. *Gastroenterology* 2006; **130**: 2031–8.

5   McMullin MF, Reilly JT, Campbell P, *et al*. Amendment to the guideline for diagnosis and investigation of polycythaemia/erythrocytosis. *Br J Haematol* 2007; **138**: 821–2.

# 24  Primary myelofibrosis

## Case History

A 54-year-old previously fit insurance salesman presents with lethargy, weight loss and night sweats. Blood tests reveal haemoglobin 7.5 g/dl, white blood cell count $19 \times 10^9$/l and platelets $846 \times 10^9$/l. The blood film is reported as being leukoerythroblastic with 2% circulating blasts; bone marrow aspirate and trephine are subsequently reported as primary myelofibrosis (PMF).

**What should the initial management plan be?**

**Is he a candidate for a bone marrow transplant?**

## Background

A leukoerythroblastic blood film, in which immature white cell precursors (including blasts) and nucleated red blood cells are seen, is highly indicative of an infiltrative process affecting the bone marrow. The differential diagnosis includes malignancy (both haematological and secondary bone marrow involvement from non-haematological malignancy), infection involving the bone marrow (for example tuberculosis) and myelofibrosis. The patient mentions a nagging abdominal pain he has had for several months and clinical examination reveals an enlarged spleen that stretches to the umbilicus. Causes of such gross splenomegaly are few, and myelofibrosis would be the most likely diagnosis. The patient underwent a bone marrow examination and the diagnosis was confirmed.

Primary myelofibrosis is a clonal myeloproliferative neoplasm characterized by the proliferation of mainly megakaryocytic and granulocytic elements in the bone marrow, associated with reactive deposition of bone marrow connective tissue (although an early pre-fibrotic phase is also recognized) and with extramedullary haematopoiesis. The incidence is approximately 1 new case per 100 000 population per year. The median age at diagnosis is 65 years, while only 22% of cases are in individuals <56 years and 11% in those <46 years. Diagnosis may follow incidental blood count abnormalities but patients may also present with symptomatic splenomegaly, constitutional symptoms, bone pain, gout secondary to hyperuricaemia or symptoms related to bone marrow failure. Most patients have splenomegaly, which may be massive, and nearly half have hepatomegaly. Most are anaemic, while platelet and leukocyte counts may be low, normal or raised. A blood film typically shows a leukoerythroblastic picture with teardrop poikilocytes. Folate levels may be low due to increased cell turnover. Median survival is 4 years but there is considerable variation between individuals. Causes of death include infection, bleeding, thrombosis (arterial/venous) or transformation to acute myeloid leukaemia, which occurs in nearly 20% of cases.[1]

Prognostic scoring systems have been used to help identify candidates for allogeneic bone marrow transplantation (alloBMT) and divide patients into low, intermediate and high risk (Table 24.1). Allogeneic BMT represents the only curative treatment and by replacing the abnormal stem cell clone with normal donor haematopoietic precursors, the stimulus for reactive marrow fibrosis is removed. For conventional myeloablative alloBMT, the transplant-related mortality (TRM) of 30% is significant, with a 5-year survival of only 30%–50%, although the majority of these patients are disease free. Better outcome has been associated with younger age, busulphan/cyclophosphamide conditioning and the absence of markers of advanced disease (e.g. absence of circulating blasts, less marrow fibrosis). A sibling donor appeared superior to an unrelated donor in some but not all studies. Pre-transplant splenectomy has been used for patients with severe marrow fibrosis or massive splenomegaly in an attempt to reduce their risk of delayed or failed engraftment. This procedure remains contentious, however, because of the operative mortality risk.

**Table 24.1 Prognostic scoring systems for PMF**

| System | Adverse factor (each scores 1) | Score | Median survival (months) | *Risk* |
|---|---|---|---|---|
| **Dupriez (Lille system)**[6] | Leukocytes <4 or >30 × 10⁹/l | 0 | 93 | Low |
| All ages, *n* = 195, median OS 42 months | Haemoglobin <10 g/dl | 1 | 26 | Intermediate |
| | | 2 | 13 | High |
| **Cervantes**[7] | Haemoglobin <10 g/dl | 0–1 | 76 | Low |
| Age ≤55, *n* = 121, median OS 128 months | Circulating blasts ≥1% | 2–3 | 33 | High |
| | Constitutional symptoms | | | |
| **Dingli**[8] | Leukocytes <4 or >30 × 10⁹/l | 0 | 155 | Low |
| Age <60, *n* = 160, median OS 78 months | Haemoglobin <10 g/dl | 1 | 69 | Intermediate |
| | Platelets <100 × 10⁹/l | 2–3 | 23.5 | High |

OS, overall survival.

The majority of cases are unsuitable for alloBMT and for these patients treatment is symptomatic and has not been shown to improve overall survival. Treatment can therefore be delayed in those who are asymptomatic at presentation.[1] Supportive care includes analgesia, replacement of haematinic deficiencies, allopurinol for hyperuricaemia, blood transfusion and appropriate involvement of palliative services. Cytotoxic therapy has a role in the proliferative phase. The most commonly used agent, hydroxycarbamide, can control leukocytosis, thrombocytosis and constitutional symptoms and reduces liver and spleen size in a significant proportion of patients. It is usually started at a low dose (e.g. 500 mg/day) as it can aggravate anaemia.[2] Low-dose melphalan and 2-chloro-deoxyadenosine (2-CDA; cladribine) are effective alternatives for control of organomegaly and thrombocytosis/leukocytosis in over half of patients treated but can cause haematological toxicity. There is also less certainty regarding their mutagenic potential. Interferon alfa is often poorly tolerated due to toxicity but may be considered for cytoreduction in refractory patients.

Androgens such as oxymetholone or the synthetic attenuated androgen, danazol, improve anaemia in 40% of cases but are less effective for patients with massive splenomegaly or abnormal cytogenetics. Fluid retention, hirsutism, deranged liver function and liver and prostate tumours have been reported. Screening for prostate cancer and abdominal ultrasound surveillance are therefore recommended.[3]

Splenectomy has been carried out for symptomatic splenomegaly, constitutional symptoms, refractory anaemia and portal hypertension. Careful case selection is essential to balance risk and benefit. Post-operative hepatic enlargement due to compensatory myeloid metaplasia occurred in 10% of cases and thrombocytosis in 29%, the latter being associated with an increased risk of thrombosis. Splenic irradiation provides symptomatic relief for a median of 6 months and can be considered in those not fit for surgery, but it can result in severe persistent cytopenias with an associated mortality rate from sepsis/haemorrhage of 13%. Deposits of extramedullary haematopoiesis can cause organ damage, peritoneal or pleural effusions and pulmonary hypertension. Deposits are sensitive to low-dose radiotherapy, which is the treatment of choice, although control is usually only temporary.

# Recent Developments

Although the aetiology of myelofibrosis remains unclear, an activating somatic point mutation in the gene encoding the cytoplasmic Janus kinase 2 ($JAK2^{V617F}$), present in around 50% of patients with PMF, has been recently discovered. It is regarded as a breakthrough as it is also present in ET and PV and appears exclusive to disorders of the myeloid lineage. It is present in stem cells of patients with PV, where it is thought to provide a proliferative advantage though activation of downstream signalling pathways. $JAK2^{V617F}$ has currently no clear prognostic value that might influence management but presents a target for novel drug agents[4] and early clinical trials of $JAK2$ inhibitors are currently underway. Somatic mutations in the thrombopoietin receptor MPL have also been found in 5–10% of patients with PMF.

Anaemia can respond to recombinant human erythropoietin (rhEPO) and response is predicted by an inappropriately low serum EPO level (<125 U/l), less severe anaemia and favourable cytogenetics. A typical starting dose is 10 000 units three times a week, doubled if no response after 1–2 months and discontinued if no response in 3–4 months.

The bisphosphonate, pamidronate, has been reported to control bone pain while zolendronate appears to reduce megakaryocyte numbers and fibrosis.

The stromal bone marrow reaction in PMF that leads to fibrosis, osteosclerosis and neoangiogenesis is driven by abnormalities of cytokines such as transforming growth factor-β, basic fibroblast growth factor and vascular endothelial growth factor. This has led to the use of the antiangiogenic and immunomodulatory drug, thalidomide, in phase II trials, with improvements in anaemia and thrombocytopenia and a reduction in splenomegaly for some patients. However, with conventional doses of 100 mg/day or more, over half of patients are intolerant, and while 50 mg/day combined with prednisolone appeared effective and better tolerated in one study, another did not show benefit of thalidomide 400 mg/day over placebo in a double-blind randomized study of 52

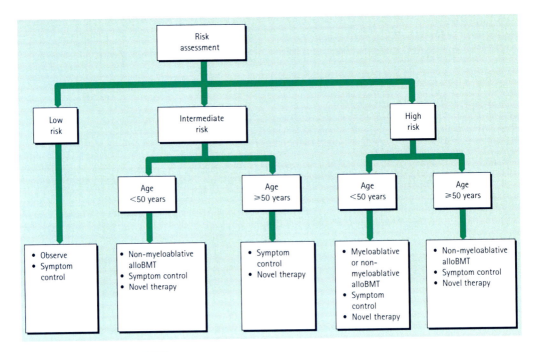

**Fig. 24.1** The treatment of PMF.

patients.[2] The more potent immunomodulatory agent, lenalidomide, appears promising in phase II trials.

Non-myeloablative alloBMT has recently been carried out, aiming to exploit the graft-versus-myelofibrosis effect while reducing the TRM. In one series, disease-free survival (DFS) was 81% at 31 months (median age 53 years, range 32–63, $n = 21$) and in another, estimated DFS was 84% at 3 years (median age 54 years, range 46–68, $n = 21$).[2] A recent series of ten patients supported these findings, with 90% of patients alive at a median of 53 months.[5] Although alloBMT offers long-term DFS for some, TRM is significant and it would be hard to justify in low-risk patients whose life expectancy would otherwise exceed 10 years (Table 24.1). The place of alloBMT is included in a suggested treatment algorithm (Figure 24.1).

## Conclusion

This patient has an intermediate (Dupriez, Dingli) or high (Cervantes) prognostic risk score and his survival is therefore likely to be less than 5 years. His blood counts suggested a proliferative stage and, in view of this, hydroxycarbamide 1 g daily together with allopurinol prophylaxis was commenced, with a reduction in his white cell count and platelets and 50% shrinkage in the size of his spleen over a period of 3 months. His iron, vitamin B12 and folate levels were normal, but serum EPO level was <125 U/l. He was therefore given a trial of rhEPO for 8 weeks, but this did not reduce his transfusion requirements, which amounted to two units every 3 weeks to relieve symptoms of anaemia. Tissue typing of his three siblings revealed one brother to be a human leukocyte antigen (HLA)-identical match and, given his poor prognosis, he was referred for alloBMT.

## Further Reading

1 Arana-Yi C, Quintás-Cardama A, Giles F, *et al.* Advances in the therapy of chronic idiopathic myelofibrosis. *Oncologist* 2006; **11**: 929–43.

2 Cervantes F. Modern management of myelofibrosis. *Br J Haematol* 2005; **128**: 583–92.

3 Reilly JT. Idiopathic myelofibrosis: pathogenesis to treatment. *Hematol Oncol* 2006; **24**: 56–63.

4 Tefferi A. Classification, diagnosis and management of myeloproliferative disorders in the JAK2V617F era. *Hematology Am Soc Hematol Educ Program* 2006: 240–5.

5 Merup M, Lazarevic V, Nahi H, *et al.* Different outcome of allogeneic transplantation in myelofibrosis using conventional or reduced-intensity conditioning regimens. *Br J Haematol* 2006; **135**: 367–73.

6 Dupriez B, Morel P, Demory JL, *et al.* Prognostic factors in agnogenic myeloid metaplasia: a report on 195 cases with a new scoring system. *Blood* 1996; **88**: 1013–18.

7 Cervantes F, Barosi G, Demory JL, *et al.* Myelofibrosis with myeloid metaplasia in young individuals: disease characteristics, prognostic factors and identification of risk groups. *Br J Haematol* 1998; **102**: 684–90.

8 Dingli D, Schwager SM, Mesa RA, Li CY, Tefferi A. Prognosis in transplant-eligible patients with agnogenic myeloid metaplasia: a simple CBC-based scoring system. *Cancer* 2006; **106**: 623–30.

# 25 Essential thrombocythaemia

## Case History

A 36-year-old pregnant woman is referred at 16 weeks gestation with a raised platelet count. Her haemoglobin level is 11.4 g/dl, white cell count $12 \times 10^9$/l and platelets $924 \times 10^9$/l. This is her first pregnancy and she has been previously fit and well.

**How would you investigate the thrombocytosis?**

## Background

The differential diagnosis (Table 25.1) is between primary and secondary causes. Pseudothrombocytosis (leukocytes/red cells misread as platelets by the automated counter) can generally be excluded on a blood film. In unselected patients attending hospital, thrombocytosis is due to reactive/secondary causes in 88%–97%. The most common secondary causes are infection, tissue damage, malignancy and chronic inflammatory disorders.[1] Since thrombocytosis can be the presenting feature of malignancy (commonly gastrointestinal, lung and lymphoma), all patients require follow-up if a cause is not identified. Weight loss, fatigue, poor appetite, night sweats, symptoms of bone marrow failure and splenomegaly suggest a primary disorder, while symptoms and signs of secondary thrombocytosis reflect the underlying cause (e.g. splenectomy scar). Those with a primary cause usually have higher platelet and leukocyte counts, haematocrit, lactate dehydrogenase (LDH) and serum potassium (pseudohyperkalaemia occurs due to leakage of intracellular potassium during blood clotting *in vitro*; a lithium–heparin/plasma sample will be more accurate). Abnormalities on the full blood count and film, in addition to thrombocytosis, suggest a primary cause and vitamin B12 may be raised (but is also elevated in liver disease, carcinoma, leukaemia and leukocytosis). Those with a secondary cause usually have a higher erythrocyte sedimentation rate (ESR) and higher fibrinogen level. Additional investigations for a secondary cause will be directed by history and examination but may include serum ferritin, antinuclear antibody (ANA) and infection screen. If a primary cause is suspected, bone marrow aspirate and trephine with cytogenetic analysis are required.

The pathogenesis of secondary thrombocytosis is not fully understood but may be mediated by thrombopoietin and pro-inflammatory cytokines such as interleukin-6. Secondary thrombocytosis does not appear to increase the risk of thrombosis unless additional risk factors are present, such as recent surgery or underlying malignancy. Primary thrombocytosis, caused by clonal stem cell abnormalities, is associated with an increase in arterial or venous thrombotic events, which are reported in 12% of patients. A

| Table 25.1 Differential diagnosis of thrombocytosis |
| --- |

**Primary thrombocytosis**

- Polycythaemia vera
- Essential thrombocythaemia
- Primary myelofibrosis
- Chronic myeloid leukaemia
- Myelodysplasia

**Secondary thrombocytosis**

- Infection (acute/chronic)
- Inflammatory disorders (e.g. systemic lupus erythematosus, Crohn's disease)
- Tissue trauma
- Fetal necrosis
- Drugs (e.g. vincristine)
- Rebound post-chemotherapy
- Hyposplenism (surgical/functional)
- Malignancy
- Iron-deficiency anaemia

**Pseudothrombocytosis** (leukocytes/red cells misread as platelets by automated counter)

- Haemoglobin H disease
- Chronic lymphocytic leukaemia
- Microspherocytosis

maternal history of unexplained abortion, stillbirth or pre-eclampsia also suggests a primary cause.

On further questioning, she has had two first-trimester miscarriages. She has no cardiovascular risk factors and no family or personal history of thrombosis. She reports a burning sensation in her feet. Her examination is unremarkable and the fetal ultrasound is normal. Blood film, ESR, ferritin, ANA and urine analysis are normal but LDH is 558 IU/l. Her bone marrow aspirate and trephine reveals changes in keeping with a diagnosis of essential thrombocythaemia.

### How would you manage her pregnancy?

Essential thrombocythaemia (ET) is a clonal myeloproliferative neoplasm attributed to transformation of a multipotent haematopoietic progenitor. The incidence is 1.5–2.5 per 100 000 per year. Patients may report microcirculatory symptoms, characteristically erythromelalgia, resulting in burning pain, warmth and redness in the extremities, which is worse in warm conditions and, in rare cases, progresses to digital necrosis and skin ulceration. Light-headedness, headaches and visual disturbances also occur. Major causes of morbidity in patients with ET are thrombosis and haemorrhage, with reported rates of 7%–17% and 8%–14%, respectively.[2] Haemorrhage is predicted by a platelet count >1000–1500 × 10$^9$/l and is due to functional platelet defects and an acquired von Willebrand's disease. Normalization of the platelet count is associated with a resolution of the bleeding tendency.[3] Thrombotic events include stroke, myocardial infarction and peripheral arterial or venous thrombosis. Risk factors for cardiovascular disease (smoking, hypertension, hypercholesterolaemia and diabetes) should therefore be aggressively controlled in all patients. Thrombotic risk is reduced by cytoreductive agents such as hydroxycarbamide and these should be used in patients who are at high risk of vascular complications, i.e. >60 years old, a platelet count >1500 × 10$^9$/l, major haemorrhage or history of thrombosis. Those aged 40–60 years have a higher thrombotic risk than those aged <40 years and familial thrombophilia also increases risk. An intermediate risk category has therefore been proposed but with variable definitions. It is unclear whether those not classed as high risk would benefit from cytoreductive therapy but this is undergoing prospective evaluation in the PT-1 trial in the UK. Aspirin is effective for microvascular symptoms and is also generally recommended for patients with prior thrombotic events in the absence of contraindications. There is no consensus for use of aspirin outside these indications, with a lack of prospective studies demonstrating benefit in ET. Aspirin as primary prophylaxis has, however, been shown to be safe and effective at reducing thrombotic events in polycythaemia vera. Essential thrombocythaemia can also transform to myelofibrosis, in around 15% of cases after 15 years, or to acute myeloid leukaemia at a rate of 0.6%–5% in 3–7 years.[2]

# Recent Developments

The outcome of over 300 pregnancies in patients with ET has been reported in the literature and an increased risk of obstetric complications has been found. A recent review excluded papers reporting fewer than five patients in order to reduce reporting bias towards negative outcome.[4] The live birth rate was 60% (full-term normal delivery rate 49%), first-trimester abortion occurred in 31% and intrauterine death or stillbirth in 6%. This must be compared with normal pregnancies in which the miscarriage rate is 10%–15% and the full-term normal delivery rate is 80%. Although normal pregnancy is associated with an increased thrombotic risk, maternal complications in ET appear to be infrequent, with a 5% risk of thrombotic events and 3% risk of major bleeding. The Janus kinase 2 mutation, present in about half of ET patients, has been reported to be an independent predictor of pregnancy complications[5] but this has yet to be confirmed in subsequent publications.

Because pregnancy in patients with ET is a rare event, most reports are retrospective, uncontrolled and non-randomized. In the absence of clear scientific evidence, guidance is based on available information and expert opinion. When pregnancy is planned in a patient known to have ET, teratogenic drugs should be stopped 3 months before conception and risk assessed through history and thrombophilia testing. Management should be risk stratified. Pregnancy can be considered high risk if there has been a prior thrombotic or major haemorrhagic event, a platelet count >1000 × 10$^9$/l or a previous severe pregnancy complication (three or more first-trimester losses or one or more second- or third-trimester losses, birth weight below the fifth centile of gestation, pre-eclampsia, intrauterine death or stillbirth). Uterine artery Doppler scanning at 20 and 24 weeks gestation can detect placental dysfunction, which predicts severe pregnancy complications,[6] and it has been suggested that the findings of an abnormal Doppler scan or two or more hereditary thrombophilic defects can also be considered high risk.[4]

Therapeutic modalities include aspirin, low-molecular-weight heparin (LMWH) and cytoreductive therapy. Aspirin has been shown to be safe in pregnancy and some but not all published data suggest a beneficial effect of low-dose aspirin (50–100 mg) in ET during pregnancy. It has been recommended for either (1) those with microvascular symptoms or a previous pregnancy complication or (2) all patients without a contraindication, e.g. prior bleeding diathesis. Care should be taken when the platelet count is >1000 × 10$^9$/l as bleeding risk is increased. Aspirin treatment should commence when the pregnancy test is positive. The addition of LMWH thromboprophylaxis for 6 weeks post-partum has been justified by reports of post-delivery microvascular complications and thrombosis in ET. Low-molecular-weight heparin has been shown to be effective prophylaxis in non-ET pregnancies where there is a high thrombotic risk. When combined with aspirin it improves the live birth rate over aspirin alone in antiphospholipid syndrome, although the pathogenesis of vascular occlusion may differ from ET. The addition of LMWH should therefore be considered in high-risk pregnancies. Discontinuation of aspirin 1–2 weeks before labour is expected and of LMWH 12 hours (if prophylactic) to 24 hours (if therapeutic) before delivery will facilitate the use of epidural analgesia. Thromboembolic deterrent stockings (TEDS) are encouraged throughout pregnancy and for 6 weeks post-partum in all ET patients. The use of plateletpheresis has been reported in a few cases but its effect is transient (usually required twice weekly) and it has a limited role, e.g. when rapid control of platelets is required or as a second-line modality. Cytoreductive therapy is controversial because, so far, no relationship has been found between platelet count and adverse pregnancy outcome. Anagrelide is not recommended in pregnancy as it crosses the placenta and can cause fetal thrombocytopenia. Hydroxycarbamide and busulphan should also be avoided due to their potential teratogenic effects. Interferon alfa does not cross the placenta and is the cytoreductive agent of choice. It appears to be excreted in breast milk and breast feeding is not recommended during treatment. Interferon alfa appears to improve pregnancy outcome, although experience is limited, and should be considered in high-risk pregnancies.

The European LeukemiaNet organization has set up a prospective, observational registry of pregnancies in chronic myeloproliferative disorders to document their course and outcome in a systematic fashion.

## Conclusion

An algorithm for management of pregnancy in ET is illustrated in Figure 25.1. The patient has microcirculatory symptoms and aspirin should be commenced. She should be encouraged to wear TEDS but since the pregnancy is not high risk, cytoreductive therapy is not required. Platelet count should be checked 4-weekly until 24 weeks and then 2-weekly. Interferon alfa should be considered if the platelet count rises above 1000 × 10$^9$/l (although in ET, platelet counts often decline spontaneously in the second trimester). Low-molecular-weight heparin should be added for 6 weeks post-delivery. Post-partum rebound thrombocytosis may need treatment with cytoreductive therapy.

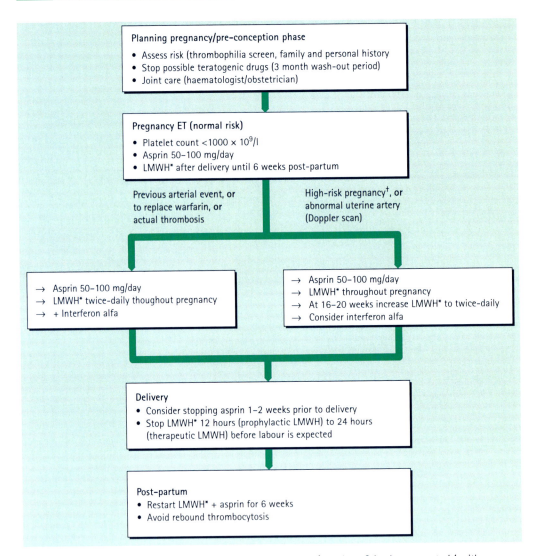

**Planning pregnancy/pre-conception phase**
- Assess risk (thrombophilia screen, family and personal history
- Stop possible teratogenic drugs (3 month wash-out period)
- Joint care (haematologist/obstetrician)

**Pregnancy ET (normal risk)**
- Platelet count <1000 × 10⁹/l
- Asprin 50–100 mg/day
- LMWH* after delivery until 6 weeks post-partum

Previous arterial event, or to replace warfarin, or actual thrombosis

High-risk pregnancy†, or abnormal uterine artery (Doppler scan)

→ Asprin 50–100 mg/day
→ LMWH* twice-daily thoughout pregnancy
→ + Interferon alfa

→ Asprin 50–100 mg/day
→ LMWH* throughout pregnancy
→ At 16–20 weeks increase LMWH* to twice-daily
→ Consider interferon alfa

**Delivery**
- Consider stopping asprin 1–2 weeks prior to delivery
- Stop LMWH* 12 hours (prophylactic LMWH) to 24 hours (therapeutic LMWH) before labour is expected

**Post-partum**
- Restart LMWH* + asprin for 6 weeks
- Avoid rebound thrombocytosis

**Fig. 25.1** Suggested management algorithm for pregnancy in ET (based on Griesshammer *et al.*,[4] with permission). *Enoxaparin 40 mg or dalteparin 5000 IU; †high-risk pregnancy: previous maternal major thromboembolic or major haemorrhagic complications, or severe complications in a previous pregnancy, or an increasing platelet count during pregnancy >1000 × 10⁹/l.

# Further Reading

1 Griesshammer M, Bangerter M, Sauer T, Wennauer R, Bergmann L, Heimpel H. Aetiology and clinical significance of thrombocytosis: analysis of 732 patients with an elevated platelet count. *J Intern Med* 1999; **245**: 295–300.

2 Finazzi G, Harrison C. Essential thrombocythemia. *Semin Hematol* 2005; **42**: 230–38.

3 Elliott MA, Tefferi A. Thrombocythaemia and pregnancy. *Best Pract Res Clin Haematol* 2003; **16**: 227–42.

4 Griesshammer M, Struve S, Harrison CM. Essential thrombocythemia/polycythemia vera and pregnancy: the need for an observational study in Europe. *Semin Thromb Hemost* 2006; **32(4 Pt 2)**: 422–9.

5 Passamonti F, Randi ML, Rumi E, *et al.* Increased risk of pregnancy complications in patients with essential thrombocythemia carrying the JAK2 (617V>F) mutation. *Blood* 2007; **110**: 485–9.

6 Harrison C. Pregnancy and its management in the Philadelphia negative myeloproliferative diseases. *Br J Haematol* 2005; **129**: 293–306.

**PROBLEM**

# 26 Hypereosinophilic syndrome

## Case History

A 25-year-old man is admitted via Accident and Emergency complaining of a 2-week history of skin rash, headache and palpitations. A full blood count reveals him to have a haemoglobin level of 13 g/dl, a raised white cell count of $28 \times 10^9/l$, with $25 \times 10^9/l$ eosinophils, and platelet count of $175 \times 10^9/l$.

**What should be your approach to investigation and management?**

## Background

This patient presents with fairly non-specific symptoms but a marked peripheral blood eosinophilia. In considering causes of eosinophilia, one first has to consider reactive causes. These may be relatively common, such as:

● a drug reaction, particularly to gold, sulphonamides and antibiotics;
● parasitic infections, including hookworm, filariasis, amoebiasis and schistosomiasis;
● atopy – asthma, eczema, etc.

Less common causes would be:

● skin diseases such as pemphigus and dermatitis herpetiformis;
● connective tissue diseases such as polyarteritis nodosa;
● lymphomas including Hodgkin lymphoma.

However, there are a number of primary causes of overproduction of eosinophils that are relatively rare but probably relevant to this case by dint of the high eosinophil count. These include:

- hypereosinophilic syndrome (HES);
- chronic eosinophilic leukaemia (CEL);
- acute myeloid leukaemia with eosinophilia (M4Eo);
- chronic myeloid leukaemia.

A full history and examination is required, particularly concentrating on drug history, history of allergic conditions and, to assess the risk of parasite infection, potential exposure during foreign travel. Clinical examination should identify evidence of dermatological disorders, connective tissue disease and lymphoproliferative disorders. Investigations should include blood film examination, stool analysis to exclude parasitic infection, skin biopsy in dermatological conditions and lymph node biopsy or bone marrow examination in suspected lymphoproliferative disorders.

The level of eosinophil count in this case means that HES or an eosinophilic leukaemia should be considered. The former can be defined as:[1]

- persistent eosinophilia of $>1.5 \times 10^9$/l for at least 6 weeks;
- lack of evidence of parasitic, allergic or other known cause;
- signs and symptoms of organ involvement.

In cases of HES, the male to female ratio is 9:1 with occurrence at a peak age of 20–50 years. The condition may be associated with significant end-organ damage particularly cardiac abnormalities. His symptoms of palpitations may be relevant in this regard.

## Organ involvement in hypereosinophilic syndrome

Clinical history and examination should identify some of the more common organ-specific syndromes associated with HES, notably cardiovascular involvement including cardiomyopathy, restrictive pericarditis, endomyocarditis and occasional mural thrombi and endomyocardial fibrosis. Patients may also give a history of dermatological abnormalities with angio-oedema, urticaria and occasionally papules, nodules and plaques. Neurological abnormalities reported include peripheral neuropathy, encephalopathy and eosinophilic meningitis; pulmonary involvement (which needs to be distinguished from asthma-related complications in reactive eosinophilia) includes pulmonary infiltrates, effusions and fibrosis. A number of other non-specific abnormalities such as hepatomegaly, eye problems including retinal arteritis and episcleritis, ascites, arthritis and bursitis, and nephrotic syndrome have all been reported. In considering gastrointestinal involvement, the absence of significant peripheral blood or bone marrow involvement would suggest an alternative diagnosis of eosinophilic gastritis/enteritis. In some cases, an abnormal proliferation of clonal T cells can be detected in the peripheral blood – so-called T-cell associated HES.

Chronic eosinophilic leukaemia, on the other hand, is a clonal proliferation of eosinophils that may be associated with an increased blast count in the peripheral blood (more than 2%) or bone marrow (5%–90%).[2] Cytogenetic abnormalities may be found and bone marrow examination would be essential in excluding this diagnosis.

Other methods of establishing clonality in CEL would include fluorescent *in situ* hybridization or assessment of X-chromosome inactivation in women, neither of which are available for routine testing. It would also be appropriate in the setting of a high blast count to exclude the subtype of acute myeloid leukaemia with eosinophilia – M4Eo in the French–American–British (FAB) classification of acute leukaemia – which is associated with a specific chromosome abnormality involving chromosome 16 (inverted 16).

Occasionally chronic myeloid leukaemia may present with a high peripheral blood eosinophil count. This diagnosis can be confirmed by the presence of the Philadelphia chromosome in cytogenetic analysis of a bone marrow sample, or by peripheral blood detection of the *BCR-ABL* oncogene by polymerase chain reaction (PCR) methodology.

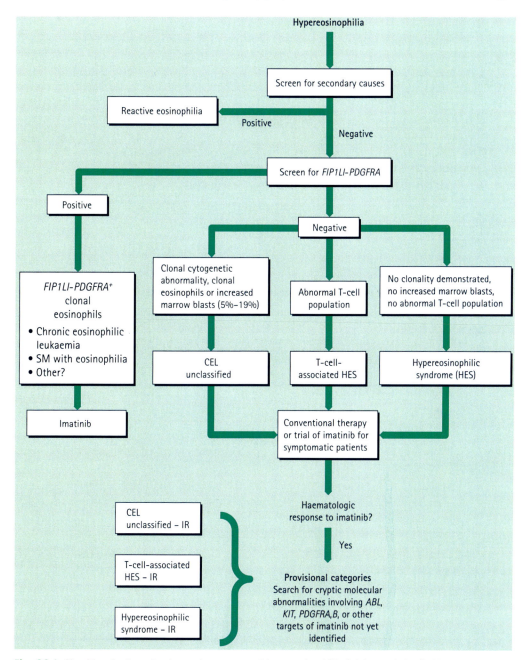

**Fig. 26.1** Algorithm for investigation and treatment of hypereosinophilia (with permission[4]). CEL, chronic eosinophilic leukaemia; HES, hypereosinophilic leukaemia; IR, imatinib-responsive; SM, systemic mastocytosis.

The recent identification of a *FIP1L1-PDGFRA* fusion gene in cases of HES allows a different approach to diagnosis and management (see Recent Developments).

## Recent Developments

It has been found that the majority of clonal proliferations of eosinophils are associated with a specific fusion protein (*FIP1L1-PDGFRA*) encoded on chromosome 4. This fusion protein predicts response to the new tyrosine kinase inhibitor, imatinib, to which HES is exquisitely sensitive, often at very low doses.[3] The chromosomal abnormality is found in approximately 50% of cases but, interestingly, even cases negative for the fusion gene may show responses to imatinib. Gotlib *et al.*[4] have proposed an algorithm to define a diagnostic and therapeutic approach to patients with persistent eosinophilia in whom reactive causes have been excluded (Figure 26.1). Conventional therapies for HES have traditionally included steroids and hydroxyurea and occasional alkalating agent therapy though the responses to this are not good.

## Conclusion

This gentleman almost certainly has HES. Peripheral blood was sent for *FIP1L1-PDGFRA* PCR to establish whether he might have *FIP1L1-PDGFRA*-positive clonal eosinophilia. The test was negative and therefore the patient was treated conventionally with oral steroids (prednisolone 1 mg/kg) rather than with a trial of imatinib therapy. His symptoms improved and the rash disappeared, which was mirrored by a fall in his eosinophil count to normal levels. Prednisolone was discontinued after 4 months but his eosinophilia and symptoms recurred after a further 18 months. He is currently receiving a clinical trial of imatinib therapy.

## Further Reading

1 Chusid MJ, Dale DC, West BC, Wolff SM. The hypereosinophilic syndrome: analysis of fourteen cases with review of the literature. *Medicine (Baltimore)* 1975; **54**: 1–27.

2 Bain B, Pierre R, Imbert M, Vardiman JW, Brunning RD, Flandrin G. Chronic eosinophilic leukaemia and the hypereosinophilic syndrome. In: Jaffe ES, Harris NL, Stein H, Vardiman JW (eds). *World Health Organization of Tumours: Tumours of Haematopoietic and Lymphoid Tissues.* Lyon, France: IARC Press, 2001; 29–31.

3 Cools J, DeAngelo DJ, Gotlib J, *et al.* A tyrosine kinase created by fusion of the PDGFRA and FIP1L1 genes as a therapeutic target of imatinib in idiopathic hypereosinophilic syndrome. *N Engl J Med* 2003; **348**: 1201–14.

4 Gotlib J, Cools J, Malone JM 3rd, Schrier SL, Gilliland DG, Coutré SE. The FIP1L1-PDGFRα fusion tyrosine kinase in hypereosinophilic syndrome and chronic eosinophilic leukemia: implications for diagnosis, classification, and management. *Blood* 2004; **103**: 2879–91.

# Lymphoma

## PROBLEM

## 27  Hodgkin lymphoma – early stage disease

## Case History

A 66-year-old man presented with a mass in the right neck. He had had this for a couple of months but it had not increased in size. He had been a smoker but had given up 5 years previously. He was otherwise fit and well apart from having had a transurethral resection of his prostate. On examination he had a 3 cm × 3 cm firm lymph node in the right mid-cervical region. There was no other palpable lymphadenopathy, hepatosplenomegaly or abnormality to be seen in the head and neck region.

**What is the differential diagnosis in this patient and what investigations should be performed to establish a diagnosis?**

## Background

In a man of this age with a node of this size the most likely cause is a malignant process. As he has been a smoker the most likely diagnosis is metastatic disease from an occult primary tumour in the upper aerodigestive tract. The other possibilities include a lymphoproliferative disease or metastatic disease from elsewhere. An infective aetiology is possible but in the absence of other symptoms or lymphadenopathy it is relatively unlikely.

Investigations should include:

- a fine needle aspirate (FNA) of the node. It is essential to establish a histological diagnosis and the patient should be referred to a head and neck surgeon with an interest in oncology;
- full blood count, which might be abnormal in infection or some lymphoproliferative diseases;
- serum urea, creatinine, electrolytes, calcium and phosphate and liver function tests. Head and neck cancer is more common in people who drink alcohol to excess;
- chest X-ray to exclude lung metastases or a primary lung cancer.

The patient attended the head and neck outpatient clinic and had a FNA performed on the lymph node. This was reported as showing no evidence of malignancy. The patient also had a fibre-optic nasoendoscopy, which did not reveal an obvious primary tumour. A computed tomography (CT) scan of the head and neck region showed no abnormality apart from the enlarged right mid-cervical lymph node. The patient was then admitted for an examination under anaesthetic and a formal lymph node biopsy.

The lymph node biopsy revealed nodular sclerosing Hodgkin lymphoma of classical variety. It is relatively common for a FNA of lymph nodes to be normal in patients with lymphoproliferative diseases (LPD) and a normal FNA does not exclude LPD. A formal biopsy, preferably with excision of the whole lymph node, is required to establish a diagnosis of lymphoma.

The patient's staging investigations were completed with a CT scan of the chest, abdomen and pelvis and a bone marrow aspirate and trephine. There was no abnormality detected on any of these investigations.

## Hodgkin lymphoma

Hodgkin lymphoma is staged using the Cotswold modification of the Ann Arbor classification (Table 27.1).[1]

The patient therefore had stage IA nodular sclerosing classical Hodgkin lymphoma. Patients with stage I and II disease have localized Hodgkin lymphoma.

Adverse prognostic indicators for patients with localized disease include age over 45 years at the time of diagnosis, being male, a raised erythrocyte sedimentation rate, haemoglobin <10.5 g/dl, lymphocytes $<0.6 \times 10^9$/l, the presence of B symptoms and extranodal sites of disease.[2] Histology is relevant, in that lymphocyte-predominant nodular Hodgkin lymphoma is a separate histological[3] and clinical entity from classical Hodgkin lymphoma. It is usually localized at presentation, managed with local radiotherapy and has a good prognosis.[4]

Finally, the patient's general health and pre-existing medical conditions may affect his or her ability to tolerate chemotherapy (see below).

The introduction of radiotherapy to the treatment of Hodgkin lymphoma offered the first chance of cure. It became clear that after treatment of the involved lymph nodes only, approximately 50% of patients would relapse in adjacent nodes. This resulted in the development of the mantle extended field radiotherapy technique, which allows all of the major lymph node groups above the diaphragm to be treated in continuity whilst mini-

**Table 27.1** Staging of Hodgkin lymphoma using the Cotswold modification of the Ann Arbor classification[1]

| Stage | Area of involvement |
|---|---|
| I | One lymph node region or one extralymphatic (E) organ or site |
| II | Two or more lymph node regions +/- one extralymphatic organ (E) on the same side of the diaphragm |
| III | Lymph node regions on both sides of the diaphragm +/- one extralymphatic organ |
| IV | One or more extralymphatic organs with or without associated lymph node involvement |

For staging purposes the spleen is considered to be a 'lymph node'.

The following are added:

B    in the presence of B symptoms, which are:
- drenching night sweats
- weight loss >10% of the body weight in the previous 6 months
- Pel Ebstein fever (recurring unexplained fever >38.5°C)

A    in the absence of B symptoms

X    if any lymph node mass is greater than 10 cm in diameter

E    in the presence of extranodal disease

mizing the radiation dose to the lungs, and inverted Y radiotherapy, which irradiates all of the major lymph node groups below the diaphragm. This development reduced the risk of relapse by approximately 11%, although no difference in overall survival is seen now as patients who relapse may be successfully salvaged with chemotherapy.[5,6]

The introduction of chemotherapy to first-line treatment offered the possibility of higher disease-free survival rates of around 90%. Through successive trials, treatment has evolved to try to offer the optimum chance of cure with a minimum of toxicity.[7,8]

# Recent Developments

Long-term toxicity is a major consideration when designing treatment schedules for Hodgkin lymphoma, which is most common in young adults and has a high cure rate. The current standard treatment for early (stage IA or non-bulky IIA) Hodgkin lymphoma is with chemotherapy plus radiotherapy to the involved nodal region (involved field radiotherapy). This minimizes the toxicity from each of these treatments by reducing the total dose of chemotherapy required and the volume of tissue that is irradiated.

The most commonly used chemotherapy is three or four cycles of ABVD (adriamycin [doxorubicin], bleomycin, vinblastine and dacarbazine) given fortnightly for 3 or 4 months. There are trials underway to determine whether the radiotherapy might be omitted from this regimen with equivalent results.

For patients who are unfit to receive ABVD chemotherapy, less intensive chemotherapy using ChlVPP (chlorambucil, vinblastine, procarbazine and prednisolone) may be used prior to involved field radiotherapy.[9] For patients unfit to receive chemotherapy, consideration should be given to treating with involved field radiotherapy only or extended field (mantle) radiotherapy, as this may cure or control the patient's disease for the duration of their life.

## Side effects – chemotherapy

ABVD may cause the following side effects.

- Nausea and vomiting, which are treated symptomatically.
- Alopecia. Hair will regrow within weeks of completion of chemotherapy.
- Myelosuppression. Neutropenia with increased risk of infection is the commonest consequence of myelosuppression. Patients must understand the need to seek urgent medical care if they develop symptoms of infection. Patients commonly require granulocyte colony-stimulating factor (G-CSF) to ensure that their blood count has recovered sufficiently to avoid delays in chemotherapy. Repeated delays in chemotherapy reduce the effectiveness of the treatment. Bone marrow reserve deteriorates with age and elderly patients are therefore more likely to develop neutropenia and sepsis as a result of chemotherapy.
- Fatigue.
- Urate release. Allopurinol should be given to reduce risk of nephropathy and acute gout.
- Infertility. ABVD is less likely to cause infertility than other chemotherapy regimens commonly used in the treatment of Hodgkin lymphoma. Male patients should be offered sperm banking. Currently, preserving primordial follicles is not widely available for women and use of this technology is still at a very early stage. Women may also undergo an early menopause as a result of chemotherapy.
- Second malignancy. This is relatively rare with this regimen compared with other regimens used to treat to Hodgkin lymphoma despite maintaining similar tumour response rates to other regimens.
- Peripheral neuropathy due to vinblastine. This is more common in elderly patients.
- Cardiomyopathy. The risk of cardiomyopathy increases with the total dose of adriamycin (doxorubicin) given. Previous cardiac problems may increase the risk of cardiomyopathy. If there is any doubt, left ventricular function should be measured prior to treatment.
- Interstitial lung disease and skin pigmentation due to bleomycin.

## Side effects – radiotherapy

The potential side effects of radiotherapy are localized to the area being treated. The risk of developing side effects increases with dose of radiotherapy delivered. As Hodgkin lymphoma is relatively radiosensitive, the dose of radiotherapy required is relatively low. For radiotherapy to one side of the neck, the possible side effects are:

- during and immediately after treatment
  - skin reaction
  - sore throat or difficulty swallowing;
- long term – these are rare but potentially serious
  - increased risk of second malignancies within the irradiated area
  - risk of osteoradionecrosis of the mandible after invasive dental procedures.

### How should this patient be treated?

Despite his age, he was fit and had no significant previous illnesses. He was, therefore, treated with 3 months of ABVD chemotherapy followed by involved field radiotherapy to the right neck. He did, however, require G-CSF support to maintain the intensity of his chemotherapy. One month after completion of chemotherapy, he received radiotherapy (30 Gy in 15 fractions) to the right side of the neck.

He tolerated the treatment well apart from suffering from fatigue. Older patients have a poorer prognosis than younger patients. This is thought to be related to them presenting more commonly with advanced disease and their poorer tolerance of chemotherapy, which may necessitate reduction in the intensity of the chemotherapy due to delays and dose reductions or the use of less toxic regimens that are less active.[10]

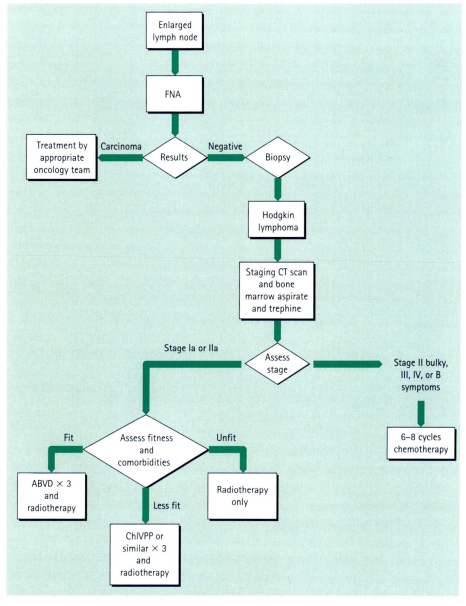

**Figure 27.1** Diagnosis and management of Hodgkin lymphoma.

# Conclusion

The long-term disease-free survival for early Hodgkin lymphoma is now greater than 90%. As this patient only had early stage disease and managed to have full-intensity treatment, he should have the same chance of disease-free survival as a younger patient. An algorithm for the diagnosis and management of Hodgkin lymphoma is shown in Figure 27.1.

# Further Reading

1 Lister TA, Crowther D, Sutcliffe SB, et al. Report of a committee convened to discuss the evaluation and staging of patients with Hodgkin's disease: Cotswolds meeting. *J Clin Oncol* 1989; **7**: 1630–36.

2 Gisselbrecht C, Mounier N, André M, et al. How to define intermediate stage in Hodgkin's lymphoma? *Eur J Haematol Suppl* 2005; (66): 111–14.

3 Jaffe ES, Harris NI, Stein H, Vardiman JW. *Pathology and Genetics: Tumours of Haematopoietic and Lymphoid Tissue*, 1st edition. Oxford: Oxford University Press, 2001.

4 Wilder RB, Schlembach PJ, Jones D, et al. European Organization for Research and Treatment of Cancer and Groupe d'Etude des Lymphomes de l'Adulte very favorable and favorable, lymphocyte-predominant Hodgkin disease. *Cancer* 2002; **94**: 1731–8.

5 Hoskin PJ, Smith P, Maughan TS, et al. Long-term results of a randomised trial of involved field radiotherapy vs extended field radiotherapy in stage I and II Hodgkin lymphoma. *Clin Oncol (R Coll Radiol)* 2005; **17**: 47–53.

6 Specht L, Gray RG, Clarke MJ, Peto R. Influence of more extensive radiotherapy and adjuvant chemotherapy on long-term outcome of early stage Hodgkin's disease: a meta-analysis of 23 randomized trials involving 3,888 patients. *J Clin Oncol* 1998; **16**: 830–43.

7 Noordijk EM, Carde P, Dupouy N, et al. Combined-modality therapy for clinical stage I or II Hodgkin's lymphoma: long-term results of the European Organisation for Research and Treatment of Cancer H7 randomized controlled trials. *J Clin Oncol* 2006; **24**: 3128–35.

8 Engert A, Schiller P, Josting A, et al. Involved-field radiotherapy is equally effective and less toxic compared with extended-field radiotherapy after four cycles of chemotherapy in patients with early-stage unfavorable Hodgkin's lymphoma: results of the HD8 trial of the German Hodgkin's Lymphoma Study Group. *J Clin Oncol* 2003; **21**: 3601–8.

9 Feltl D, Vítek P, Zámecnïk J. Hodgkin's lymphoma in the elderly: the results of 10 years of follow-up. *Leuk Lymphoma* 2006; **47**: 1518–22.

10 Engert A, Ballovam V, Haverkamp H, et al. Hodgkin's lymphoma in elderly patients: a comprehensive retrospective analysis from the German Hodgkin's Study Group. *J Clin Oncol* 2005; **23**: 5052–60.

# 28 Hodgkin lymphoma – advanced stage disease and long–term sequelae

## Case History

A 34-year-old woman presented with a dry cough for some weeks and feeling intermittently that her voice had changed. The only other symptom that she volunteered was that she had noticed increasing itching over the previous 6 months. On questioning she admitted to losing 6 kg in weight in the last few months without trying and that she woke up at night sweating two or three times a week. She had no other symptoms of note. She had no significant past medical history and took no regular medication. She lived with her husband and two sons aged 5 and 8 years. They had no pets. She did not smoke. On examination there were no abnormal signs; in particular, she was apyrexial, had no palpable lymph nodes and her chest was clear. Her blood tests, including a full blood count, urea, electrolytes, calcium and phosphate, and liver function tests, were all normal, apart from a mildly raised plasma viscosity. A chest X-ray showed mediastinal widening.

**What is the most likely diagnosis and what further investigations should be arranged?**

## Background

The differential diagnosis in a young woman is:

- malignancy;
- tuberculosis;
- sarcoidosis.

A computed tomography (CT) scan would be helpful in assessing the cause of the mediastinal widening and excluding the presence of a lung parenchymal abnormality that might be associated with tuberculosis.

In this patient the CT scan confirmed the presence of lymphadenopathy from the left lower-cervical region extending through the mediastinum to the subcarinal lymph nodes. The largest lymph node mass was 5 cm × 8 cm at the level of the aortic arch. There were no abnormalities in the lung parenchyma.

Lymphadenopathy this extensive is most likely to be due to malignancy. The most likely malignancy in a young woman with no significant past medical history and who is a non-smoker is a lymphoma. Drenching night sweats are a recognized symptom of lymphoma, as is itching, although the latter is relatively rare.

A mediastinal biopsy was performed. This showed nodular sclerosing Hodgkin lymphoma. Staging investigations were completed with a CT scan of the abdomen and pelvis and a bone marrow aspirate and trephine test. These showed no evidence of disease.

The presence of night sweats, weight loss of >10% of the body weight in the previous 6 months or Pel Ebstein fever are B symptoms, which have an adverse prognostic significance. It should be noted that itching does not constitute a B symptom. The disease is staged according to the Ann Arbor classification. She has stage IIB disease, i.e. disease confined to lymph nodes on one side of the diaphragm (*see* Table 27.1).

Combination chemotherapy is the treatment of choice in Hodgkin lymphoma for patients with B symptoms, bulky lymphadenopathy or stage III or IV disease, i.e. advanced disease. These patients usually receive a minimum of six cycles of chemotherapy. Various chemotherapy combinations have been used in the past but ABVD (adriamycin [doxorubicin], bleomycin, vinblastine and dacarbazine) has generally become the treatment of choice.[1,2] ABVD has the advantages of causing less infertility and having a lower rate of second malignancy compared with the other equipotent regimens. The 5-year progression-free survival rate for patients treated with ABVD is approximately 75%.

The German Hodgkin Study Group's BEACOPP regimen (bleomycin, etoposide, adriamycin [doxorubicin], cyclophosphamide, vincristine, procarbazine and prednisolone) showed an improved 5-year relapse-free survival when compared with COP-PABVD (cyclophosphamide, vincristine, procarbazine, prednisolone and ABVD).[3] The incidences of second malignancies, particularly leukaemia, and infertility are significantly higher after treatment with BEACOPP as compared with ABVD. It has been suggested that BEACOPP should be reserved for patients with a poorer prognosis. The Hasenclever index can be used to determine prognosis in advanced Hodgkin lymphoma. It identifies seven adverse prognostic factors:

- >45 years of age;
- male sex;
- serum albumin <40 g/l;
- haemoglobin <10.6 g/l;
- stage IV disease;
- white cell count <15.0 × 10$^9$/l;
- lymphocyte count <0.6 × 10$^9$/l.

The presence of each of these reduces the chance of disease-free survival at 5 years by 8%.[4] It has been suggested that patients with four or more adverse prognostic factors might be considered for more intensive therapy than ABVD.

The patient was treated with ABVD. Clinically, the itching and night sweats subsided as the disease responded. A repeat CT scan after three cycles showed that the patient had had a good partial response but repeat scanning showed no further significant improvement after six cycles. There was discussion about whether the patient would benefit from adjuvant radiotherapy to the mediastinum at the end of chemotherapy and whether positron emission tomography (PET) scanning would be helpful in determining optimum treatment.

## Recent Developments

 It has been shown that there is no place for adjuvant radiotherapy after chemotherapy in patients who have achieved a complete response, i.e. with no evidence of residual abnormality on CT scanning at the end of chemotherapy.[5] The use of adjuvant radiotherapy at the end of chemotherapy for patients with residual abnormalities on CT scanning is more controversial because:

● it has never been shown to improve overall survival, as patients who relapse can be salvaged with high-dose chemotherapy and autologous stem cell transplantation. Radiotherapy may, however, improve relapse-free survival;
● there is an increased risk of patients developing second cancers within the irradiated area. These are usually solid tumours. They start to occur approximately 10 years after the radiotherapy and their incidence increases with time. Evidence does, however, suggest that the patients requiring second-line chemotherapy may be at the greatest risk for second cancers;[6]
● there is particular concern about the risk of breast cancer in women under the age of 30 years at the time of radiotherapy to the mediastinum or axillae. For smokers, there is a high risk of developing secondary lung cancer after mediastinal radiotherapy;
● radiotherapy to the mediastinum is associated with an increased risk of cardiac problems, especially for patients who smoke.[7]

It is common for patients with Hodgkin lymphoma to have residual abnormalities in the mediastinum on completion of chemotherapy. Until recently there was no accurate method of determining whether the mass contained active tumour, but this has changed with the advent of $^{18}$F-fluoro-deoxyglucose PET (FDG-PET) scanning.

## FDG–PET scanning

Whereas CT scanning demonstrates anatomical abnormalities, PET scans give functional information about the abnormalities. Positron emission tomography scanning is reported to have a specificity of >90% and false-negative rate of 10% in staging Hodgkin lymphoma. It is also being used increasingly to assess response to treatment. It has been suggested that patients who have a negative PET scan at the end of chemotherapy, even where the CT scan demonstrates residual abnormality, have a very low chance of relapse.

Further studies have suggested that PET scans should be performed before treatment starts and after two cycles of chemotherapy; 90% of patients whose PET scan is negative after two cycles of chemotherapy remain in remission 2 years after completion of treatment, whereas 90% of patients who have a positive PET scan after two cycles of chemotherapy develop progressive disease within 2 years.[8] It has been suggested that the outcome of a PET scan after two cycles of chemotherapy could be used to intensify or reduce patients' chemotherapy. Clinical trials are underway to test this hypothesis.

At the end of treatment, the patient's PET scan was positive and further assessment with CT scanning showed unequivocal evidence of disease progression, with an increase in size of the mediastinal mass. The patient also developed night sweats again.

**What should the treatment approach now be?**

The patient is relapsing.

● Fit patients should be treated with a relapse chemotherapy schedule. These are more intensive than ABVD and usually contain cisplatinum in combination with other drugs, e.g. etoposide and cytarabine or dexamethasone and cytarabine. It is usual to give two to four cycles of chemotherapy followed by peripheral blood stem cell (PBSC) harvest, then high-dose chemotherapy using BEAM (carmustine, etoposide, cytarabine and melphalan) with PBSC rescue. The overall 5-year survival for this treatment is 50%.[9] Patients who progress during first-line treatment or who have had multiple previous chemotherapy regimens do less well than those with first relapse more than a year after completion of first-line treatment.

● Even patients who do not respond to relapse chemotherapy schedules may still benefit from a BEAM autograft,[10] although patients who respond to second-line chemotherapy prior to transplant do have a better prognosis than those who do not.

● For patients who are not suitable for an autograft, with an isolated relapse, wide field or involved field radiotherapy should be considered.[11]

● For patients who relapse after all of the above, and who are still candidates for active treatment, a non-myeloablative allogeneic stem cell transplant should be considered.

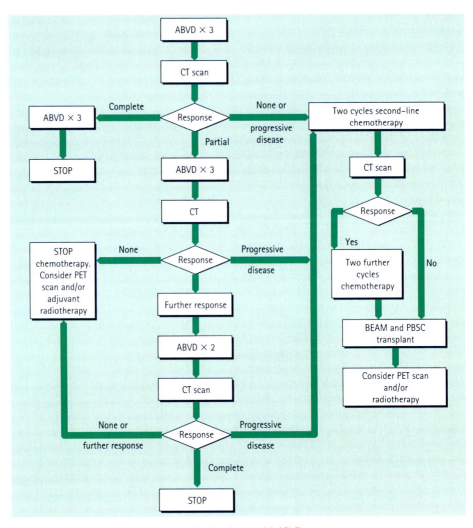

**Figure 28.1** Treatment of advanced Hodgkin lymphoma with ABVD.

## Conclusion

The patient went on to have four cycles of cisplatinum-based chemotherapy with a good response, then a BEAM autograft followed by mediastinal radiotherapy. Her PET scan on completion of treatment was negative. She remains well with no evidence of relapse 18 months after completion of chemotherapy. A flow diagram outlining the treatment of advanced Hodgkin lymphoma is shown in Figure 28.1.

## Further Reading

1 Gobbi PG, Levis A, Chisesi T, *et al.* ABVD versus modified stanford V versus MOPPEBVCAD with optional and limited radiotherapy in intermediate- and advanced-stage Hodgkin's lymphoma: final results of a multicenter randomized trial by the Intergruppo Italiano Linfomi. *J Clin Oncol* 2005; **23**: 9198–207.

2 Johnson PWM, Radford JA, Cullen MH, *et al.* Comparison of ABVD and alternating or hybrid multidrug regimens for the treatment of advanced Hodgkin's lymphoma: results of the United Kingdom Lymphoma Group LY09 Trial. *J Clin Oncol* 2005; **23**: 9208–18.

3 Diehl V, Franklin J, Pfreundschuh M, *et al.* Standard and increased-dose BEACOPP chemotherapy compared with COPP-ABVD for advanced Hodgkin's disease. *N Engl J Med* 2003; **348**: 2386–95.

4 Hasenclever D, Diehl V. A prognostic score for advanced Hodgkin's disease. International Prognostic Factors Project on Advanced Hodgkin's Disease. *N Engl J Med* 1998; **339**: 1506–14.

5 Laskar S, Gupta T, Vimal S, *et al.* Consolidation radiation after complete remission in Hodgkin's disease following six cycles of doxorubicin, bleomycin, vinblastine, and dacarbazine chemotherapy: is there a need? *J Clin Oncol* 2004; **22**: 62–8.

6 Franklin J, Pluetschow A, Paus M, *et al.* Second malignancy risk associated with treatment of Hodgkin's lymphoma: meta-analysis of the randomised trials. *Ann Oncol* 2006; **17**: 1749–60.

7 Swerdlow AJ, Higgins CD, Smith P, *et al.* Myocardial infarction mortality risk after treatment for Hodgkin disease: a collaborative British cohort study. *J Natl Cancer Inst* 2007; **99**: 206–14.

8 Gallamini A, Rigacci L, Merli F, *et al.* The predictive value of positron emission tomography scanning performed after two courses of standard therapy on treatment outcome in advanced stage Hodgkin's disease. *Haematologica* 2006; **91**: 475–81.

9 Lavoie JC, Connors JM, Phillips GL, *et al.* High-dose chemotherapy and autologous stem cell transplantation for primary refractory or relapsed Hodgkin lymphoma: long-term outcome in the first 100 patients treated in Vancouver. *Blood* 2005; **106**: 1473–8.

10 Tarella C, Cuttica A, Vitolo U, *et al.* High-dose sequential chemotherapy and peripheral blood progenitor cell autografting in patients with refractory and/or recurrent Hodgkin lymphoma: a multicenter study of the Intergruppo Italiano Linfomi showing prolonged disease free survival in patients treated at first recurrence. *Cancer* 2003; **97**: 2748–59.

11 Josting A, Nogová L, Franklin J, *et al.* Salvage radiotherapy in patients with relapsed and refractory Hodgkin's lymphoma: a retrospective analysis from the German Hodgkin Lymphoma Study Group. *J Clin Oncol* 2005; **23**: 1522–9.

**PROBLEM**

# 29 High-grade diffuse large B-cell non-Hodgkin lymphoma

## Case History

A 29-year-old woman presents to her doctor in the 30th week of a previously normal pregnancy. She has recently noticed some chest discomfort and a progressive feeling of swelling and tightness in her face. On examination she has obvious lymphadenopathy in the neck and signs of early superior vena cava obstruction (SVCO). A neck node is biopsied under local anaesthetic and proves to be a diffuse large B-cell non-Hodgkin lymphoma (DLBCL).

**How does the pregnancy affect the approach to investigating and staging the disease?**

**What are the options for managing the patient's lymphoma at 30 weeks of pregnancy?**

**What are her outcomes and what future therapy is available should she relapse?**

## Background

Non-Hodgkin lymphoma (NHL) is a broad term encompassing many distinct lymphoid malignancies. The histological classification is complex, but clinically there remains a working distinction between aggressive and indolent forms of the disease. Diffuse large B-cell non-Hodgkin lymphoma represents about 30% of NHLs and is the commonest aggressive lymphoma. It classically affects lymph nodes, spleen, liver or bone marrow but not infrequently spreads to other viscera, skin or the central nervous system (CNS). Initial investigation requires a good-quality biopsy and detailed staging procedures, which always include clinical history and examination, blood tests, computed tomography scanning (chest, abdomen and pelvis) and examination of the bone marrow. The lactate dehydrogenase (LDH) level is a useful marker of DLBCL; a raised level has prognostic significance at diagnosis and can be a sign of relapse during follow-up. These elements of diagnosis and staging produce clinical and laboratory information that has been used to construct prognostic scores for DLBCL, the most validated of which is the International Prognostic Index (IPI).[1] Depending on the number of risk factors the patient has at diagnosis, their anticipated 5-year survival ranges from 26% to 73%. The IPI risk factors, prognostic groups and outcomes are shown in Figure 29.1. It should be noted that age alone (below or above 60 years) is the most powerful single predictor.

**Risk factors:**

The patient scores 1 for the presence of each of the following, giving them a total of 0–5

- Patient age                              >60 years
- Disease stage                           III or IV
- Performance status                  2 or greater
- LDH                                          Above the normal limit
- Number of extranodal disease sites    More than one

**IPI score and prognostic groups:**

The score from 0–5 for the above factors defines four groups as follows:

- 0 or 1          Low risk
- 2               Low intermediate risk
- 3               High intermediate risk
- 4 or 5          High risk

**5-year survival for the prognostic groups (%):**

- Low risk                         73
- Low intermediate risk       51
- High intermediate risk      43
- High risk                        26

**Figure 29.1** The International Prognostic Index: risk factors, prognostic groups and survival (adapted with permission[1]).

First-line treatment is chemotherapy based although some elderly individuals with early stage disease may do well with local radiotherapy. In the UK, the standard of care is the administration of six to eight courses of CHOP (cyclophosphamide, adriamycin [doxorubicin], vincristine and prednisolone) chemotherapy at 21-day intervals with the addition of an infusion of the anti-CD20 monoclonal antibody rituximab with each of the courses. This combination is referred to as R-CHOP21.[2] For early (localized) disease, the number of courses of R-CHOP21 may be reduced to three and radiation given to the area involved. This produces excellent results and minimizes toxicity. Attempts to intensify front-line chemotherapy have met with limited success and greater toxicity and CHOP has stood the test of time in this respect.[3] Recent modifications to the timing of the schedule may, however, be of value (see below). A further complicating issue in planning treatment is the possibility of CNS involvement. This is more likely in those with higher IPI scores or a raised LDH level and is also a feature of disease in certain specific sites (e.g. the sinuses). It is quite rare at diagnosis but seen at relapse in 5% of cases. If this is an issue then, in addition to the standard therapy described above, CNS-penetrating chemotherapy must be given. This is conventionally methotrexate by the intrathecal route but recent practice is moving to high-dose intravenous infusions of this drug, which achieve superior drug levels in the brain and cerebrospinal fluid.

Relapse of DLBCL is a serious problem and although further chemotherapy is often effective and can produce some long-term survivors, most will die of their disease. For those who are younger and fitter, peripheral blood stem cell transplantation (a form of dose escalation) has been shown to be effective and may rescue up to 50% of patients.[4]

# Recent Developments

### 1. The use of rituximab

This monoclonal antibody has an established place in the therapy of B-cell NHL in many settings. It is directed at a B-cell antigen (CD20) and antibody binding leads to malignant (and normal) B-cell depletion. It is an effective single agent in low-grade NHL, has shown excellent results in combination with standard chemotherapy in low- and high-grade disease and may have a further role as a maintenance agent.[5,6] In DLBCL, the combination of rituximab and CHOP has demonstrated the first consistent improvement in overall survival for many years – and with no added toxicity.[2]

### 2. Increasing dose intensity (R–CHOP14)

Growth factor support (with granulocyte colony-stimulating factor) shortens the neutropenic period after chemotherapy, allowing R-CHOP to be given every 14 days instead of every 21 days. Trials of this approach, which have been performed with and without rituximab, suggest that R-CHOP14 may be a new standard for therapy and this has been adopted in many European countries. Ongoing trials in the UK will help to confirm this and may change our practice.[7]

### 3. Allogeneic bone marrow transplantation

Improvements in the safety and understanding of this procedure have led to studies in lymphomas of a 'graft-versus-lymphoma' effect, i.e. a donor-derived immune response against residual lymphoma in the patient after they receive the donor marrow. Results are quite preliminary and mainly in heavily pretreated patients to date, but such manoeuvres may prove useful in younger patients in the future and offer a chance of cure.[8]

#### How does this patient's pregnancy affect her management?

The presentation is due to large nodes in the neck and mediastinum causing incipient SVCO. The patient is 30 weeks pregnant – potentially deliverable but with significant risk to the child from prematurity and to her from the delivery. Computed tomography or radiography are contraindicated but magnetic resonance imaging can be used if imaging is essential. Staging will thus be incomplete, which may complicate decisions. Superior vena cava obstruction is likely to ensue rapidly in this case so temporizing is not an option. Such circumstances require close and detailed discussion between the patient, the haematologist and the obstetrician. The patient's own clinical risk and their personal wishes will be paramount in deciding how to proceed. Options here include a trial of steroids or commencing standard chemotherapy (R-CHOP21) with the baby *in situ*. In either case, steroids are involved and will assist lung maturity in the baby pre-delivery. If steroids alone are chosen initially, close monitoring is needed as the mother's condition could become critical if the disease response is limited. It should be borne in mind that delivery will probably be by caesarean section and it is difficult to give chemotherapy within 2 weeks of surgery. Control of the disease for a reasonable time is therefore needed (perhaps 4–6 weeks) to allow the baby to mature and the mother to recover. This may be asking a lot of steroids and argues for initial use of chemotherapy. Despite the perceived risks of chemotherapy, there is substantial evidence that it is relatively safe to both mother and child in late pregnancy and may be the best option in this case.[9,10]

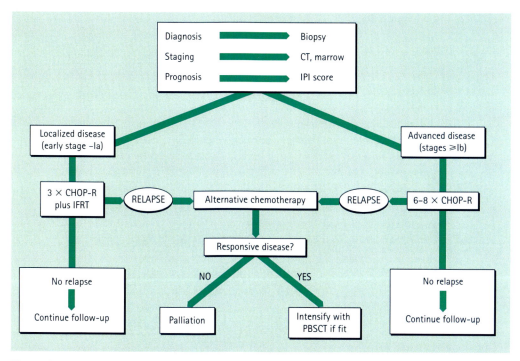

**Figure 29.2** Algorithm for the therapy of newly presenting DLBCL. The decision to intensify with peripheral blood stem cell transplantation (PBSCT) depends on patient age and fitness, with less fit subjects completing alternative chemotherapy and then being followed up. In selected younger patients, consideration of an allograft may be made as discussed in the text. CT, computed tomography; IFRT, involved field radiotherapy.

# Conclusion

DLBCL is a heterogeneous disorder and careful assessment of patient and disease-specific factors at the outset is needed to guide therapy and estimate prognosis. The attempts to improve conventional chemotherapy approaches have met with limited success but the monoclonal antibodies, particularly rituximab, have made a real impact on survival. An algorithm for the therapy of newly presenting DLBCL is shown in Figure 29.2.

# Further Reading

1 The International Non-Hodgkin's Lymphoma Prognostic Factors Project. A predictive model for aggressive non-Hodgkin's lymphoma. *N Engl J Med* 1993; **329**: 987–94.

2 Coiffier B, Lepage E, Briere J, *et al.* CHOP chemotherapy plus rituximab compared with CHOP alone in elderly patients with diffuse large-B-cell lymphoma. *N Engl J Med* 2002; **346**: 235–42.

3 Fisher RI, Gaynor ER, Dahlberg S, *et al.* Comparison of a standard regimen (CHOP) with three intensive chemotherapy regimens for advanced non-Hodgkin's lymphoma. *N Engl J Med* 1993; **328**: 1002–6.

4 Philip T, Guglielmi C, Hagenbeek A, *et al.* Autologous bone marrow transplantation as compared with salvage chemotherapy in relapses of chemotherapy-sensitive non-Hodgkin's lymphoma. *N Engl J Med* 1995; **333**: 1540–45.

5 Marcus R, Imrie K, Belch A, *et al.* CVP chemotherapy plus rituximab compared with CVP as first-line treatment for advanced follicular lymphoma. *Blood* 2005; **105**: 1417–23.

6 Forstpointner R, Unterhalt M, Dreyling M, *et al.* Maintenance therapy with rituximab leads to a significant prolongation of response duration after salvage therapy with a combination of rituximab, fludarabine, cyclophosphamide, and mitoxantrone (R-FCM) in patients with relapsed and refractory follicular and mantle cell lymphomas: results of a prospective randomized study of the German Low Grade Lymphoma Study Group (GLSG). *Blood* 2006; **108**: 4003–8.

7 Pfreundschuh M, Trümper L, Kloess M, *et al.* Two-weekly or 3-weekly CHOP chemotherapy with or without etoposide for the treatment of elderly patients with aggressive lymphomas: results of the NHL-B2 trial of the DSHNHL. *Blood* 2004; **104**: 634–41.

8 Doocey RT, Toze CL, Connors JM, *et al.* Allogeneic haematopoietic stem-cell transplantation for relapsed and refractory aggressive histology non-Hodgkin lymphoma. *Br J Haematol* 2005; **131**: 223–30.

9 Avilés A, Neri N. Hematological malignancies and pregnancy: a final report of 84 children who received chemotherapy in utero. *Clin Lymphoma* 2001; **2**: 173–7.

10 Pohlman B, Macklis RM. Lymphoma and pregnancy. *Semin Oncol* 2000; **27**: 657–66.

# 30 Primary central nervous system lymphoma

## Case History

A man aged 50 years is brought to Accident and Emergency having apparently experienced a fit while shopping. He gives a history of occasional headaches over the past few weeks and some intermittent double vision in the last week. On examination, he has a right sixth nerve palsy but is fully orientated. His family, however, report some changes in his behaviour in the last month and were becoming concerned. He had made an appointment with his General Practitioner for the following day. A computed tomography (CT) scan of his head shows a single 3 cm lesion in the left frontal lobe with some mass effect. Neurosurgical biopsy gives a histological diagnosis of diffuse large B-cell lymphoma. There is no evidence of lymphoma in any other anatomical site.

**How does one arrive at the diagnosis of primary central nervous system lymphoma (PCNSL)?**

**What biological and patient factors may influence the prognosis and management plan?**

**What are the issues in deciding on the optimum treatment for this patient?**

## Background

Primary central nervous system (CNS) lymphoma is a distinctive form of the commonest high-grade type of non-Hodgkin lymphoma (NHL) – diffuse large B-cell lymphoma. It is unusual in being entirely localized to the CNS, in contrast to systemic high-grade NHL, which is often disseminated at diagnosis. There is thus a paradox: NHL presenting outside the CNS may spread to it but PCNSL does not become systemic. There is no clear biological explanation for this.

Primary CNS lymphoma is rare but on the increase. Recent UK figures report an incidence of 2.8 per million. It may account for up to 5% of primary brain tumours. The increasing incidence appears real and is not explained by improved diagnostics or by the human immunodeficiency virus (HIV) epidemic.

It presents as a space-occupying lesion in the CNS, with or without features of meningeal involvement (e.g. cranial nerve palsies). The clinical history is short. Personality changes and cognitive impairment are common. Focal neurological impairment such as hemiparesis and aphasia is also frequently seen. Seizures occur in approximately 10%–20% of patients. Headache is rarely a prominent complaint. Radiology reveals a mass lesion which is multifocal in over a third of cases.[1] A diffuse brain abnormality with no mass lesion is also recognized and histologically there is often evidence of disease in brain tissue distant from the principal site. Primary CNS lymphoma is frequently not suspected on the basis of its radiological appearance, which may closely mimic the appearance of other CNS tumours.

Diagnosis usually requires a brain biopsy but this may be avoided if there is clear evidence on an examination of cerebrospinal fluid (CSF). Lumbar puncture is therefore essential (unless contraindicated) and is positive in 20% of cases,[1] although autopsy studies suggest that unrecognized meningeal involvement is more common.[2] Involvement of the ocular structures is detected by slit-lamp examination in 15% of cases. By definition, routine staging tests to detect lymphoma outside the CNS must be negative, so CT scan-

---

**1. Required initial tests for diagnosis, staging and prognostic scoring:**

| Test | Notes |
|---|---|
| • MRI of brain | CT less informative |
| • Brain biopsy | Neurosurgical – often stereotactic |
| • CSF examination | Morphology, flow cytometry, protein assay |
| • Ocular examination | Slit-lamp examination of the ocular fundus |
| • Staging CT scan | Encompassing chest, abdomen, pelvis |
| • Bone marrow examination | Rarely positive if staging CT is clear |
| • HIV serology | Increased incidence of PCNSL in acquired immune deficiency syndrome |
| • Lactate dehydrogenase (LDH) | Possible prognostic value (see below) |

**2. Prognostic scoring systems and outcome**

**Ferreri et al. (2003):[5]**
Based on the following five factors (1 point for each):

- Age >60 years
- Performance status >1
- Raised serum LDH
- Raised CSF protein
- Tumour involvement of deep brain matter

Derived from a retrospective analysis of 378 immunocompetent PCNSL patients treated at 23 centres. Patients were grouped as high (score 4–5), medium (score 2–3) or low risk (score 0–1). Two-year overall survival rates were 15% ± 7%, 48% ± 7% and 80% ± 8%, respectively.

**Bessell et al. (2004) (Nottingham/Barcelona scoring system):[12]**
Based on the following three factors (1 point for each):

- Age ≥60 years
- Performance status ≥2
- Extent of disease (multifocal vs unifocal)

Derived from 77 patients with PCNSL treated with combination chemotherapy and WBRT. Median survival durations were 55, 41, 32 and 1 month for scores of 0, 1, 2 and 3, respectively.

**Note:**
Other analyses have found age >60 years and poor performance status to be important but failed to define other factors.

**Figure 30.1** Diagnosis, staging and prognostic factors in PCNSL – key points. MRI, magnetic resonance imaging; WBRT, whole brain radiotherapy.

ning (chest, abdomen and pelvis) and a bone marrow examination are carried out. These initial procedures are summarized in Figure 30.1.

Prognosis in PCNSL is a difficult subject and published series give very different figures as a consequence of their diverse patient selection. Historically, when treatment was with whole brain radiotherapy (WBRT) alone, the prognosis was dismal, with median survival of 12 months and <10% of patients attaining a good long-term outcome.[3] Many patients are elderly and frail and the neurological dysfunction they present with limits the prognostic outlook. A retrospective series of 55 consecutively diagnosed cases underlined this, with 45% of patients being deemed unfit to receive any but simple palliative therapy.[4] However, for those who are fit, the most successful chemotherapy regimens achieve a median survival of up to 60 months with an estimated 30%–40% long-term survival.[1] Age and performance status appear to be the main determinants of prognosis. Several groups have analysed other factors and attempted to produce a reliable prognostic scoring system but the rarity of the disease and variability of outcome have made this task complex.[5] Possible prognostic models are shown in Figure 30.1.

Therapy for PCNSL used to be a simple (if depressing) subject for the reasons outlined above. The blood–brain barrier prevented almost all the accepted antilymphoma drugs from reaching the tumour unless injected directly into the CSF by lumbar puncture. This was the reason for a reliance on radiotherapy. Experimental efforts to chemically disrupt this barrier and allow drug passage were largely unhelpful. In recent years, however, it has proved possible to deliver a number of effective drugs (principally high-dose methotrex-

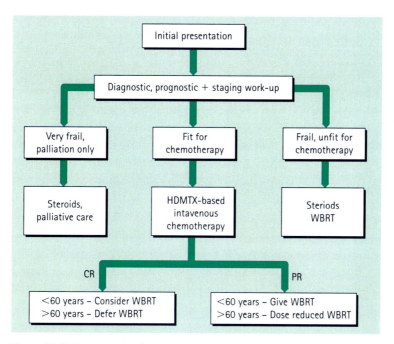

**Figure 30.2** Treatment algorithm for newly presenting PCNSL. Note: decisions regarding the use of WBRT following intravenous chemotherapy are complex and remain contentious, as outlined in the main text. More trial evidence is required to inform the balance between disease control and long-term neurotoxicity before practice can be standardized. The flow chart shown is only one suggested guide. CR, complete remission; PR, partial remission.

ate [HDMTX]) intravenously at doses that penetrate the CNS and produce tumouricidal drug levels.[6] This has made the most significant impact on the outcome of PCNSL so far. Intrathecally administered drugs are often still used but their value is now questionable. Recent therapies are discussed in the following section and an algorithm for treatment is presented in Figure 30.2. It needs to be appreciated that little randomized data are available and the condition is rare, so many treatment assumptions are pragmatic and based on poor levels of evidence.

# Recent Developments

### 1. The introduction of systemic chemotherapy

High-dose methotrexate is the most important agent and is effective against the tumour when given intravenously at high doses (at least 1 g/m² and up to >10 g/m²). There is much debate about the required dose needed to penetrate the CNS and whether there is a further dose response if that is escalated.[6] Further studies are needed to answer these questions. Numerous trials have shown that the addition of HDMTX to WBRT increases median survival from around 12 months to 32–60 months.[7,8] A number of other drugs have now been used in this way, including cytarabine, nitrosureas, topotecan, ifosfamide and steroids. It seems logical to treat PCNSL with combination therapy as this has become the clear standard in other lymphoma types but this approach remains intuitive rather than evidence based. Some randomized trials are in progress comparing single and combination chemotherapy but most data on these drugs are from phase II, single-arm studies.

### 2. Re-evaluation of the role of radiotherapy

With the development of effective systemic chemotherapy, there is a need to re-evaluate the role of radiotherapy. The main issue is the long-term neurological toxicity which is seen when WBRT and HDMTX are combined. This is often fatal and is reported to affect at least 20%–30% of cases, with an even higher incidence in older (>60 years) patients.[7,9] Study data are contradictory regarding the importance of WBRT if effective chemotherapy is given. The impression is that WBRT improves control but this may not be the case for the most effective chemotherapy.[7,10] The improvement is outweighed by toxicity in some studies and an important goal of research is to limit (or exclude) WBRT from treatment schedules without compromising efficacy.

### 3. The use of rituximab

This antibody is now so ubiquitous in B-cell lymphoma treatment that it deserves mention here. The pharmacology suggests that it does not achieve useful CSF levels when given intravenously and is unlikely to be efficacious. This has led to some anecdotal reports of intrathecal use, with some apparent responses.[11] Further evaluation is needed.

#### How should the patient be managed?

This man is less than 60 years old and generally fit. He should receive treatment based around HDMTX. Options include the use of HDMTX (4–6 cycles) alone followed by consideration of WBRT (taking into account the toxicity issues discussed above) or the addition of other CNS-penetrating drugs. The latter approach would be best in the context of a clinical trial as there is little evidence to guide the choice of drug at present. The aim is to achieve clinical and radiological remission. If the response is complete, serious thought should be given to avoiding WBRT as toxicity rates are high. Given the current levels of evidence, it is more difficult to defer the radiotherapy if the response is suboptimal but lower doses may be an option to consider.

## Conclusion

The patient achieved a complete response to a combination of idarubicin, dexamethasone, cytarabine and HDMTX ('IDARAM') given as part of a clinical trial. After detailed discussions on the risks and benefits of WBRT, he declined the latter. He remains alive and well and in clinical and radiological complete remission 18 months following the completion of therapy.

## Further Reading

1 DeAngelis LM. Primary central nervous system lymphomas. *Curr Treat Options Oncol* 2001; **2**: 309–18.

2 Onda K, Wakabayashi K, Tanaka R, Takahashi H. Intracranial malignant lymphomas: clinicopathological study of 26 autopsy cases. *Brain Tumor Pathol* 1999; **16**: 29–35.

3 Nelson DF. Radiotherapy in the treatment of primary central nervous system lymphoma (PCNSL). *J Neurooncol* 1999; **43**: 241–7.

4 Hodson DJ, Bowles KM, Cooke LJ, *et al.* Primary central nervous system lymphoma: a single-centre experience of 55 unselected cases. *Clin Oncol (R Coll Radiol)* 2005; **17**: 185–91.

5 Ferreri AJM, Blay JY, Reni M, *et al.* Prognostic scoring system for primary CNS lymphomas: the International Extranodal Lymphoma Study Group experience. *J Clin Oncol* 2003; **21**: 266–72.

6 Hiraga S, Arita N, Ohnishi T, *et al.* Rapid infusion of high-dose methotrexate resulting in enhanced penetration into cerebrospinal fluid and intensified tumour response in primary central nervous system lymphomas. *J Neurosurg* 1999; **91**: 221–30.

7 Abrey LE, Yahalom J, DeAngelis LM. Treatment for primary CNS lymphoma: the next step. *J Clin Oncol* 2000; **18**: 3144–50.

8 DeAngelis LM, Seiferheld W, Schold SC, Fisher B, Schultz CJ. Combination chemotherapy and radiotherapy for primary central nervous system lymphoma: Radiation Therapy Oncology Group Study 93-10. *J Clin Oncol* 2002; **20**: 4643–8.

9 Omuro AM, Ben-Porat LS, Panageas KS, *et al.* Delayed neurotoxicity in primary central nervous system lymphoma. *Arch Neurol* 2005; **62**: 1595–600.

10 Ferreri AJ, Reni M, Pasini F, *et al.* A multicenter study of treatment of primary CNS lymphoma. *Neurology* 2002; **58**: 1513–20.

11 Schulz H, Pels H, Schmidt-Wolf I, Zeelen U, Germing U, Engert A. Intraventricular treatment of relapsed central nervous system lymphoma with the anti-CD20 antibody rituximab. *Haematologica* 2004; **89**: 753–4.

12 Bessell EM, Graus F, Lopez-Guillermo A, *et al.* Primary non-Hodgkin's lymphoma of the CNS treated with CHOD/BVAM or BVAM chemotherapy before radiotherapy: long-term survival and prognostic factors. *Int J Radiat Oncol Biol Phys* 2004; **59**: 501–8.

# 31 Indolent lymphoma – follicular non-Hodgkin lymphoma

## Case History

A 66-year-old man was diagnosed with follicular lymphoma 6 years ago. He responded well to oral chlorambucil chemotherapy. Four years later, his disease recurred and he received intravenous combination chemotherapy along with the therapeutic antibody rituximab.

**What prognostic features are useful in planning therapy in this disease?**

## Background

Follicular lymphoma (FL) is a low-grade malignancy and is the second commonest type of non-Hodgkin lymphoma (NHL). Its incidence increases with age.[1]

Presentation is usually with asymptomatic lymphadenopathy but patients may have systemic symptoms such as weight loss, fevers, lethargy or night sweats. The bone marrow may be involved with resulting cytopenias. Most patients present at an advanced stage because the disease develops slowly with few symptoms, but localized disease is sometimes seen and this has a good outlook. The behaviour of FL, although indolent in most cases, is variable and there is a significant risk (around 2%–3% per year) of transformation to a histologically aggressive large-cell NHL.[2]

Diagnosis is usually made from histology of lymph node, bone marrow or other tissue and is supported by the finding of a typical t(14;18) chromosomal translocation. Staging investigations include a computed tomography scan of the neck, chest, abdomen and pelvis and a bone marrow biopsy.

Follicular lymphoma is not curable, with the debatable exception of localized (stage Ia) presentations. For most patients, the disease course is characterized by responses to treatment followed by observation, relapse and further therapy. Subsequent responses tend to be of shorter duration and the median overall survival is 10 years. A significant minority will transform to high-grade NHL, a situation which has a poor outlook.[2]

A useful prognostic score has been designed employing five risk factors, which are readily available at diagnosis (Table 31.1). This score, the Follicular Lymphoma International Prognostic Index (FLIPI), is useful in the design of studies that stratify therapy according to patient risk group. It can also help clinicians to decide whether more intensive therapy is justified for some patients.[3] Three risk groups are identified according to the number of risk factors from the FLIPI, with 5-year survival rates ranging from 52% to 90% (Table 31.2).

| Table 31.1 The Follicular Lymphoma International Prognostic Index (FLIPI) | |
|---|---|
| Parameter | Adverse factor |
| Age≥60 years | |
| Ann Arbor stage | III–IV |
| Haemoglobin level | <120 g/l |
| Serum LDH level | >Upper normal limit |
| Number of nodal sites | >4 |

The five factors in this table are combined to produce a score (0–4), which assigns the patient to a prognostic group as shown in Table 31.2. LDH, lactate dehydrogenase.

| Table 31.2 Assigning risk groups using the FLIPI and the impact on survival | | |
|---|---|---|
| Risk group | Number of adverse prognostic factors | Five-year survival |
| Low | 0–1 | 90.6% |
| Intermediate | 2 | 77.6% |
| High | >3 | 52.5% |

## The approach to therapy

The small number of patients who present with localized (Ann Arbor stage Ia) disease are treated with involved field radiotherapy and have an excellent long-term survival, probably equating to a cure for some.

In more advanced disease, it is important to consider the age and fitness of the patient alongside the symptoms the disease is giving them. If asymptomatic, it is reasonable to adopt a 'watch-and-wait' policy, initiating treatment only when there is evidence of symptomatic progression or deteriorating organ function. Overall survival is not altered by this conservative approach and treatment is, after all, not curative.[4]

When treatment is needed, oral chlorambucil remains valuable for some older patients but most patients are offered combination chemotherapy, usually containing steroids, vincristine and cyclophosphamide with or without an anthracycline or related agent (e.g. doxorubicin or mitoxantrone).[5,6] In recent years, it has been established that the addition of rituximab (a monoclonal anti-B-cell antibody) to these combinations is highly beneficial and this has now become the standard of care for initial therapy.[7]

Fludarabine, a purine analogue, has also been widely used. There may be a synergistic effect with fludarabine and cyclophosphamide and these agents are often combined.[8] A possible drawback with fludarabine is its association with poor cell yields when harvesting stem cells in patients eligible for autologous stem cell transplantation.

There are therefore a number of well-tried combination chemotherapy regimens, all benefiting from the addition of rituximab, but with no clear randomized data available to choose between them. If the patient has had a long initial response to treatment, the same regimen may be used again when the disease recurs, but the common practice is to change therapy, particularly if relapse is within a year. Localized relapses can be treated with radiotherapy.

After a further two years he re-presents with weight loss, night sweats and lymphadenopathy in cervical and abdominal regions. A repeat biopsy confirms follicular lymphoma.

**What are the merits of intensive therapy (autologous stem cell transplantation)?**

**What other options are available to him now?**

Intensifying therapy is a contentious issue. It is usually achieved using peripheral blood stem cell transplantation (PBSCT) and is practical up to around 60 years of age. There are few comparative data to show that this procedure is more effective than chemotherapy but a reasonable, non-randomized body of evidence suggests that fitter patients achieve good responses and their survival may be prolonged.[9] The only curative treatment available is allogeneic bone marrow transplantation. This should be considered in all young patients, especially those with aggressive disease, and is usually performed at or beyond the second relapse. The morbidity and mortality of this procedure are considerable but long-term survival may be achieved.

Patients who undergo high-grade transformation of their disease are treated as for aggressive B-cell NHL, often with CHOP (cyclophosphamide, doxorubicin, vincristine and prednisolone) plus rituximab chemotherapy and a PBSCT depending on their age. Good results can be obtained but the outcome is poor for the majority. Treatment opinion does vary between clinicians. Each case needs to be assessed individually, factoring comorbidity, age (both biological and actual) and informed patient choice.

# Recent Developments

### 1. Monoclonal antibodies

The development of these agents has dramatically changed the treatment of FL. Rituximab is a monoclonal antibody directed against B cells (recognizing the CD20 antigen on their surface). It is thought to act in several ways: complement-induced lysis, induction of apoptosis and antibody-dependent cell killing. In combination with conventional chemotherapy regimens, it greatly improves response rates and progression-free survival.[7] More recently, compelling evidence has emerged to support its use as a maintenance agent in both first remission and after relapse, the antibody being given alone at intervals over a 2-year period following chemotherapy. Striking improvements in progression-free survival have been reported in randomized trials and an overall survival advantage has now been demonstrated.[10] Some patients with advanced FL may be unsuitable for chemotherapy and rituximab can be used alone with a response in up to 50% of cases, giving useful palliation.

### 2. Radioimmunotherapy

This approach utilizes a monoclonal antibody bound to a radioisotope and is a novel approach to treating FL. The specificity of the antibody targets the radioisotope to the tumour cells thus delivering high local doses of radiation to them but a low total body dose. Ibritumomab tiuxetan is an example of such an agent. It is a conjugate of an anti-CD20 monoclonal antibody and the isotope yttrium-90 – a pure β-emitter. It is a simple, one-off administration with minimal radioprotection issues. It has been shown to be effective in patients treated with multiple chemotherapy regimens and published response rates are of the order of 70%, with some patients achieving durable long-term remissions.[11]

## Conclusion

This man is probably not a realistic candidate for intensive therapy, which is in any case contentious. He has had two forms of chemotherapy over 6 years, including rituximab. He has advanced disease and is symptomatic, so therapy seems indicated. One option is further conventional chemotherapy with rituximab, perhaps using a fludarabine and cyclophosphamide combination. Consideration would have to be given to using rituximab as maintenance afterwards and this is becoming routine practice. A reasonable alternative at this point would be to use radioimmunotherapy. This is simple and relatively non-toxic and he would still be able to have the above chemotherapy at the time of a later relapse.

## Further Reading

1 The Non-Hodgkin's Lymphoma Classification Project. A clinical evaluation of the International Lymphoma Study Group classification of non-Hodgkin's lymphoma. *Blood* 1997; **89**: 3909–18.

2 Plancarte F, López-Guillermo A, Arenillas L, *et al.* Follicular lymphoma in early stages: high risk of relapse and usefulness of the Follicular Lymphoma International Prognostic Index to predict the outcome of patients. *Eur J Haematol* 2006; **76**: 58–63.

3 Solal-Céligny P, Roy P, Colombat P, *et al.* Follicular Lymphoma International Prognostic Index. *Blood* 2004; **104**: 1258–65.

4 Ardeshna KM, Smith P, Norton A, *et al.* Long-term effect of a watch and wait policy versus immediate systemic treatment for asymptomatic advanced-stage non-Hodgkin lymphoma: a randomised controlled trial. *Lancet* 2003; **362**: 516–22.

5 Hoppe RT, Kushlan P, Kaplan HS, Rosenberg SA, Brown BW. The treatment of advanced stage favorable histology non-Hodgkin's lymphoma: a preliminary report of a randomized trial comparing single agent chemotherapy, combination chemotherapy, and whole body irradiation. *Blood* 1981; **58**: 592–8.

6 Peterson BA, Petroni GR, Frizzera G, *et al.* Prolonged single-agent versus combination chemotherapy in indolent follicular lymphomas: a study of the cancer and leukaemia group B. *J Clin Oncol* 2003; **21**: 5–15.

7 Marcus R, Imrie K, Belch A, *et al.* CVP chemotherapy plus rituximab compared with CVP as first-line treatment for advanced follicular lymphoma. *Blood* 2005; **105**: 1417–23.

8 Forstpointner R, Dreyling M, Repp R, *et al.* The addition of rituximab to a combination of fludarabine, cyclophosphamide, mitoxantrone (FCM) significantly increases the response

rate and prolongs survival as compared with FCM alone in patients with relapsed and refractory follicular and mantle cell lymphomas: results of a prospective randomized study of the German Low-Grade Lymphoma Study Group. *Blood* 2004; **104**: 3064–71.

9 Sebban C, Mounier N, Brousse N, *et al.* Standard chemotherapy with interferon compared with CHOP followed by high-dose therapy with autologous stem cell transplantation in untreated patients with advanced follicular lymphoma: the GELF-94 randomized study from the Groupe d'Etude des Lymphomes de l'Adulte (GELA). *Blood* 2006; **108**: 2540–44.

10 van Oers MH, Klasa R, Marcus RE, *et al.* Rituximab maintenance improves clinical outcome of relapsed/resistant follicular non-Hodgkin lymphoma in patients both with and without rituximab during induction: results of a prospective randomized phase 3 intergroup trial. *Blood* 2006; **108**: 3295–301.

11 Witzig TE, Gordon LI, Cabanillas F, *et al.* Randomized controlled trial of yttrium-90-labeled ibritumomab tiuxetan radioimmunotherapy versus rituximab immunotherapy for patients with relapsed or refractory low-grade, follicular, or transformed B-cell non-Hodgkin's lymphoma. *J Clin Oncol* 2002; **20**: 2453–63.

# 32 Indolent lymphoma – Waldenström's macroglobulinaemia epistaxis

## Case History

A 63-year-old man with a past history of ischaemic heart disease, diabetes and hypertension presented to his local Accident and Emergency department with a severe nose bleed. He also gave a 6-month history of intermittent headache, dizziness and blurring of vision. He was admitted by the ear, nose and throat surgeons but his nose bleeding proved difficult to control with local measures. Initial investigations revealed the following: haemoglobin 7.3 g/dl, white cell count $5.2 \times 10^9/l$ with a normal differential and platelet count $97 \times 10^9/l$. The blood film demonstrated marked rouleaux formation and his plasma viscosity was grossly elevated at 10.3 mPa.s. Renal and hepatic function were essentially normal but serum protein electrophoresis demonstrated an immunoglobulin M (IgM) κ paraprotein level of 75 g/l. This was not associated with any reduction in the levels of IgG or IgA but κ light chains were present in the urine at low concentrations. Serum $\beta_2$-microglobulin was elevated at 5 mg/l. Bone marrow examination demonstrated extensive infiltration by small lymphocytes showing plasmacytoid differentiation and a striking increase in reactive mast cells. The infiltrate had the following immunophenotype: CD5–, CD10–, CD19+, CD20+, CD22+, CD23–, CD79+, surface IgM κ+. A diagnosis of Waldenström's macroglobulinaemia (WM) was made.

**What would be your initial management plan and chemotherapeutic options?**

**What are the known prognostic factors in this disorder?**

## Background

Waldenström's macroglobulinaemia is a relatively rare B-cell lymphoproliferative disorder, which is characterized primarily by bone marrow infiltration and IgM paraproteinaemia.[1] It accounts for approximately 2% of all haematological malignancies. In the USA the annual incidence is 6.1 per million in white males and 2.5 per million in white females, although the incidence appears to be lower in non-Caucasians. In the UK the annual incidence is 10.3 per million while the median age at presentation is 71 years and the median overall survival is 60 months.[2, 3] The presenting clinical features of WM are highly variable.[2, 4, 5] Some patients are asymptomatic at presentation and are found to have an IgM paraprotein as a coincidental finding during unrelated clinical investiga-tions.[5, 6] Patients with symptomatic disease may present with features attributable to tis-sue infiltration such as anaemia, systemic symptoms and organomegaly. A proportion of patients present with clinical features directly attributable to the physicochemical prop-erties of their IgM paraprotein. These features include hyperviscosity syndrome (see below), cryoglobulinaemia and amyloidosis. The IgM paraprotein may also have autoan-tibody specificity, which can result in a number of autoimmune phenomena such as peripheral neuropathy, cold agglutinin disease, immune thrombocytopenia, acquired von Willebrand's disease and C1 esterase inhibitor deficiency (Caldwell syndrome).

Waldenström's macroglobulinaemia is characterized by bone marrow infiltration by small lymphocytes showing plasma cell differentiation. The pattern of infiltration is dif-fuse or interstitial and a reactive increase in mast cells is also a highly characteristic fea-ture.[1, 5]

### Initial management and chemotherapeutic options

The patient described in this report has hyperviscosity syndrome and should undergo urgent plasma exchange. Hyperviscosity syndrome occurs in up to 10% of patients pre-senting with WM and is characterized by fatigue, visual disturbances, headache, mucocu-taneous bleeding and heart failure. Fundoscopic abnormalities are common in such patients and comprise dilation of retinal veins, retinal haemorrhages and exudates and ultimately papilloedema.[7] The plasma viscosity at which symptoms are noted varies con-siderably from patient to patient but remains remarkably constant within individual patients. Symptoms are only rarely evident at viscosities of less than 4 mPa.s but some patients are asymptomatic with viscosities of 8 mPa.s and upwards.[7] Exchanging 1–1.5 times the calculated plasma volume is recommended in the treatment of hyperviscosity and one to two procedures appears to reduce the plasma viscosity to near-normal levels in most patients.[3] Chemotherapy should be instituted as soon as is practicable but addi-tional plasma-exchange procedures may be necessary depending upon the rate of reaccu-mulation of paraprotein. A minority of patients with refractory disease may be managed with regular exchange procedures. Blood transfusions should be avoided in the acute set-ting as they may exacerbate the hyperviscosity.

A significant minority of patients with WM (25%) are asymptomatic at presentation and do not therefore require any specific therapy.[5, 6] The majority of these patients may be monitored in the outpatient clinic at 3- to 6-monthly intervals. The overall rate of pro-gression is relatively low with a median time to progression of almost 5 years.[6] Indications for therapy in WM include haematological suppression, constitutional symptoms and bulky nodal and splenic disease. Phenomena attributable to the parapro-tein such as hyperviscosity syndrome and the autoimmune disorders are also clear indi-cations to initiate therapy.[8] Single-agent chlorambucil is effective in patients with WM as responses are seen in approximately 60% of patients. This is simple oral therapy, which is generally well tolerated by the majority of patients.[3, 9] The principal toxicities are haema-tological but responses may be slow. Purine analogues such as fludarabine and cladribine are also appropriate primary therapy in patients with WM.[3, 9] They are both, however, associated with more myelosuppression and infection risk than chlorambucil. Fludarabine is available as an oral preparation but it should be given with caution to patients with mild to moderate renal impairment (the dose should be reduced by 50% if the creatinine clearance is 30–70 ml/min and it is contraindicated if the creatinine clearance is <30ml/min). It is associated with autoimmune haemolysis in a small minority of patients. It is not clear, however, whether the purine analogues are superior to alkylating agents, although this is being assessed in an ongoing clinical trial (www.waldenstroms.org). There is no clear evidence to support the use of combination therapy such as CVP (cyclophosphamide, vincristine and prednisolone) or CHOP (cyclophosphamide, doxorubicin, vincristine and prednisolone) as primary therapy in patients with symptomatic WM.[3]

# Recent Developments

## Diagnosis

Recent studies have demonstrated that WM is characterized in most cases by a surface IgM (sIgM)[+], surface IgD[+/–], CD5–, CD10–, CD19[+], CD20[+], CD22[+], CD23–, CD25[+], CD27[+], CD75–, CD79[+], CD103–, CD138–, FMC7[+], BCL-2[+], BCL-6–, PAX-5[+] immunophenotype.[5, 10] These data were incorporated into more stringent diagnostic criteria published in 2003 and the recently revised WHO classification of haematological neoplasms.[1, 11] It is not, however, necessary to routinely assess the expression of all these antigens, as in practice a sIgM[+], CD5–, CD10–, CD19[+], CD20[+], CD23– immunopheno-type in association with a non-paratrabecular pattern of infiltration is usually diagnostic of WM.[5]

## Treatment

The monoclonal anti-CD20 antibody rituximab has recently been shown to be active in patients with WM, with responses documented in up to 50% of patients.[12] It is an attractive alternative to myelosuppressive agents but responses are frequently slow. It should be avoided (as a single agent) in patients with symptomatic hyperviscosity and those with a paraprotein concentration of greater than 40 g/l as the response rates in these groups of patients are very low and there is a significant risk of a sudden and paradoxical increase in IgM levels, which may be associated with significant morbidity and even mortality. This phenomenon has been termed 'IgM flare'. More recently, the proteasome inhibitor bortezomib has shown encouraging activity in WM. Responses in up to 60% of patients have been reported in relapsed/refractory disease.[13] Principal toxicities are thrombocytopenia, neuropathy, diarrhoea and fatigue.

## Prognostic factors

Waldenström's macroglobulinaemia, in common with other indolent lymphoproliferative disorders, has a highly variable clinical outcome. A significant minority of patients remain asymptomatic and never require therapy while others have advanced lymphoma.

Recently, an international collaborative group has proposed an International Prognostic Scoring System for WM.[14] In this analysis, five adverse prognostic factors were identified: age >65 years, haemoglobin <11.5 g/dl, platelet count <100 × 10⁹/l, $\beta_2$-microglobulin >3 mg/l and paraprotein concentration >70 g/l. In this scheme, low risk is defined as zero or one adverse features (excluding age), high risk by three or more adverse features and intermediate risk by the presence of two adverse features or age >65 years. Low-, intermediate- and high-risk features are identified in 27%, 38% and 35% of patients and are associated with 5-year survival rates of 87%, 68% and 36%, respectively.

The patient described in this case would be considered to have high-risk disease on the basis of the presence of four of the five adverse prognostic factors.

## Epidemiology and genetic factors

A number of recent studies have demonstrated that first degree relatives of WM patients have an increased risk of developing WM and its putative precursor IgM monoclonal gammopathy of undetermined significance. Additionally there appears to be an excess risk of developing other B cell disorders such as chronic lymphocytic leukaemia and non-Hodgkin lymphoma as well as quantitative abnormalities in polyclonal immunoglobulin suggesting there may a number of common susceptibility genes that predispose to WM and other lymphoproliferative disorders.[15, 16] Furthermore there is emerging data on the role of chronic antigen stimulation in the development of WM.[16] An excess risk of WM is conferred by a history of hepatitis C, human immunodeficiency virus and rickettsial infection as well as a personal history of autoimmune disease.

The patient's symptoms settled with plasma exchange and he was commenced on chlorambucil chemotherapy. He required repeated plasma exchange during the first 4 months of chemotherapy but ultimately received 12 courses of chlorambucil. At the end of this treatment his full blood count was normal and bone marrow examination showed only minimal involvement by monoclonal B cells. Approximately 3 years later he was noted to have a rising IgM level and plasma viscosity along with progressive anaemia. Bone marrow examination confirmed disease progression.

### What are the treatment options for this relapse?

Waldenström's macroglobulinaemia is not curable with conventional chemotherapeutic approaches and many patients have a relapsing and remitting course and ultimately receive many lines of therapy. Patients who achieve a durable remission (typically at least one year) with their primary therapy may be retreated with the same agent.[3, 9] In practice, the majority of patients who progress following treatment with an alkylating agent go on to receive a purine analogue. Fludarabine appears to be superior to combination therapy with CAP (cyclophosphamide, adriamycin [doxorubicin] and prednisolone) in this setting.[17]

Purine analogues and alkylating agents are known to be synergistic. Highly encouraging data are now emerging with the fludarabine–cyclophosphamide combination. Similarly, combinations of fludarabine–rituximab, both with and without cyclophosphamide, also appear highly efficacious. Likewise, combinations of cladribine and cyclophosphamide, both with and without rituximab, appear highly active in patients with WM.[18] Some caution is, however, required as there is some emerging data that suggests that purine analogue-based therapies may be associated with a higher incidence of secondary myelodysplasia / acute myeloid leukaemia and large cell transformation.[19]

There are also some data demonstrating the efficacy of thalidomide (either alone or in combination with dexamethasone and clarithromycin or rituximab), lenalidomide and alemtuzumab in patients with relapsed/refractory disease. There is as yet no clear role for stem cell transplantation, either autologous or allogeneic, in this disorder.

## Conclusion

The patient received oral fludarabine therapy, with achievement of a further remission after six courses. No further plasmapheresis was required. He continues to be monitored on a 3-monthly basis in the clinic setting. At each clinic visit the following parameters are assessed: full blood count, renal function, plasma viscosity and serum concentration of the IgM paraprotein.

## Further Reading

1 Owen RG, Treon SP, Al-Katib A, *et al.* Clinicopathological definition of Waldenstrom's macroglobulinemia: consensus panel recommendations from the Second International Workshop on Waldenstrom's Macroglobulinemia. *Semin Oncol* 2003; **30**: 110–15.

2 Dimopoulos MA, Panayiotidis P, Moulopoulos LA, Sfikakis P, Dalakas M. Waldenström's macroglobulinemia: clinical features, complications, and management. *J Clin Oncol* 2000; **18**: 214–26.

3 Johnson SA, Birchall J, Luckie C, Oscier DG, Owen RG. Guidelines on the management of Waldenström macroglobulinaemia. *Br J Haematol* 2006; **132**: 683–97.

4 Garcia-Sanz R, Montoto S, Torrequebrada A, *et al.* Waldenström macroglobulinaemia: presenting features and outcome in a series with 217 cases. *Br J Haematol* 2001; **115**: 575–82.

5 Owen RG, Barrans SL, Richards SJ, *et al.* Waldenström macroglobulinemia. Development of diagnostic criteria and identification of prognostic factors. *Am J Clin Pathol* 2001; **116**: 420–8.

6 Kyle RA, Benson J, Larson D, *et al.* IgM monoclonal gammopathy of undetermined significance and smoldering Waldenström's macroglobulinemia. *Clin Lymphoma Myeloma* 2009; **9**: 17–18.

7 Stone MJ. Waldenström's macroglobulinemia: Hyperviscosity syndrome and cryoglobulinemia. *Clin Lymphoma Myeloma* 2009; **9**: 97–99.

8 Kyle RA, Treon SP, Alexanian R, *et al.* Prognostic markers and criteria to initiate therapy in Waldenström's macroglobulinemia: consensus panel recommendations from the Second International Workshop on Waldenström's Macroglobulinemia. *Semin Oncol* 2003; **30**: 116–120.

9 Dimopoulos MA, Gertz MA, Kastritis E, *et al.* Update on treatment recomendations from the Fourth International Workshop on Waldenström's Macroglobulinemia. *J Clin Oncol* 2009; **27**: 120–6.

10 San Miguel JF, Vidriales MB, Ocio E, *et al.* Immunophenotypic analysis of Waldenström's macroglobulinemia. *Semin Oncol* 2003; **30**: 187–95.

11 Swerdlow SH, Campo E, Harris NL, *et al.* (eds). *WHO Classification of Tumours of Haematopoietic and Lymphoid Tissues.* IARC: Lyon 2008.

12 Dimopoulos MA, Kastritis E, Roussou M, *et al.* Rituximab-based treatments in Waldenström's macroglobulinemia. *Clin Lymphoma Myeloma* 2009; **9**: 59–61.

13 Chen C, Kouroukis CT, White D, *et al.* Bortezomib in relapsed or refractory Waldenström's macroglobulinemia. *Clin Lymphoma Myeloma* 2009; **9**: 74–6.

14 Morel P, Duhamel A, Gobbi P, *et al.* International Prognostic Scoring System for Waldenström's macroglobulinemia. *Blood* 2009; **113**: 4163–70.

15 McMaster ML, Kristinsson SY, Turesson I, *et al.* Novel aspects pertaining to the relationship of Waldenström's macroglobulinemia, IgM monoclonal gammopathy of undetermined significance, polyclonal gammopathy, and hypoglobulinemia. *Clin Lymphoma Myeloma* 2009; **9**: 19–22.

16 Kristinsson SY, Koshiol J, Goldin LR, *et al.* Genetics- and immune-related factors in the pathogenesis of lymphoplasmacytic lymphoma / Waldenström's macroglobulinemia. *Clin Lymphoma Myeloma* 2009; **9**: 23–6.

17 Leblond V, Levy V, Maloisel F, *et al.* Multicenter, randomized comparative trial of fludarabine and the combination of cyclophosphamide-doxorubicin-prednisone in 92 patients with Waldenström macroglobulinemia in first relapse or with primary refractory disease. *Blood* 2001; **98**: 2640–44.

18 Tedeschi A, Miqueleiz Alamos S, Ricci F, *et al.* Fludarabine-based combination therapies for Waldenström's macroglobulinemia. *Clin Lymphoma Myeloma* 2009; **9**: 67–70.

19 Leleu X, Tamburini J, Roccaro A, *et al.* Balancing risk versus benefit in the treatment of Waldenström's macroglobulinemia patients with nucleoside analogue-based therapy. *Clin Lymphoma Myeloma* 2009; **9**: 71–3.

# Plasma Cell Disorders

**PROBLEM**

# 33 Myeloma – diagnosis and prognosis

## Case History

A 62-year-old female attends a General Practitioner's surgery with a 4-week history of lower back pain, tiredness and lethargy. Initial investigations reveal a normochromic, normocytic anaemia with haemoglobin 10.4 g/dl and a raised plasma viscosity at 2.1.

**What further investigations would be indicated for the diagnosis of multiple myeloma?**

**Which parameters should be assessed to appropriately stage this myeloma?**

## Background

Plasma cell myeloma (PCM; multiple myeloma) is a plasma cell tumour with an incidence of 3–4 new cases per 100 000 population per year and accounts for approximately 10% of haematological malignancies. Patients usually present with a monoclonal band on protein electrophoresis. Most (60%) are immunoglobulin G (IgG) subclass and approximately 15% are IgA, with IgM, IgD and IgE accounting for less than 2% of patients. Occasionally there is a monoclonal excess of light chains only (approximately 20% of patients have κ or λ light chains) and in approximately 1% the myeloma is non-secretory without any serum or urinary evidence of excess antibody or light chain production.

Owing to increased awareness of the disease and availability of rapid biochemical analysis, less than 40% of patients now present with symptomatic bone disease and at least

20% of patients are now diagnosed whilst totally asymptomatic. Patients may present with hyperCalcaemia, Renal dysfunction, Anaemia, Bone fractures or lytic lesions (CRAB) but also with recurrent bacterial infections, signs and symptoms of spinal cord compression, features suggestive of amyloidosis or a persistently raised erythrocyte sedimentation rate, plasma viscosity or serum paraprotein detectable on routine investigations. Less than 10% of patients present with symptoms of hyperviscosity syndrome, which is most likely to occur in patients with IgA subclass variant. Bleeding defects also occur in approximately 15% of patients with IgG subclass and 30% of patients with IgA subclass.[1]

Initial investigations of a patient suspected of suffering from PCM should include serum and concentrated urine electrophoresis followed by immunofixation to confirm and type the monoclonal protein (paraprotein, M-protein). Quantification should be performed by electrophoretic densitometry of the monoclonal peak. Urinary light chain quantification can be performed either on a 24-hour urinary collection or on a random urinary sample calibrated in relation to the urinary creatinine level (protein creatinine index [PCI]). More recently, serum free light chain excess production (FLC assay) has been used as an alternative methodology in patients with light chain disease or those who have non-secretory disease.[2]

Bone marrow aspiration for the examination of the marrow morphology can confirm the diagnosis of myeloma (plasma cell infiltrate >10%) and a trephine biopsy should be performed at diagnosis as it provides a suitable baseline measurement to determine response to therapy (Figure 33.1). Malignant plasma cells can be differentiated from normal plasma cells by flow cytometry by the surface phenotype CD19– CD45– CD56[plus] CD138[plus]. The role of conventional metaphase cytogenetics or fluorescent *in situ* hybridization to determine clonal genetic abnormalities is currently under investigation.

A skeletal survey of the axial skeleton should be part of the initial staging process. This standard radiological imaging technique will allow large areas to be examined for generalized bone density (to detect osteopenia/osteoporosis) and lytic lesions (Figure 33.2) and assessment of the threat of pathological fractures in involved bones. In addition, any area of bone-associated pain should be imaged for distal skeletal involvement. Computed tomography has a higher sensitivity than plain radiographs at detecting small lytic lesions and can accurately depict the presence and extent of associated soft tissue infiltration. Magnetic resonance imaging is extremely useful for examining the extent and the nature of soft tissue involvement, especially for the investigation of those presenting with neurological symptoms. Positron emission tomography has recently been reported as a useful imaging technique for assessing occult disease and soft tissue infiltration. Bone scintigraphy has no routine role in the diagnosis and follow-up assessment of patients with myeloma due to its low sensitivity as a result of the lack of osteoblastic activity.

The diagnosis is usually confirmed by demonstrating the presence of a monoclonal antibody in the serum and/or urine, lytic bone lesions and an increased number of plasma cells infiltrating the bone marrow. As monoclonal antibodies are detected in other plasma cell dyscrasias (monoclonal gammopathy of undetermined significance [MGUS], amyloid, solitary plasmacytomas), an international working group has developed a classification based on the level of paraprotein, the percentage of marrow infiltration and the presence or absence of myeloma-related organ and/or tissue impairment (ROTI). The criteria define the classification of MGUS and asymptomatic and symptomatic myeloma (Figure 33.3). Patients with asymptomatic myeloma do not require treatment but do require intensive monitoring and follow-up.[1]

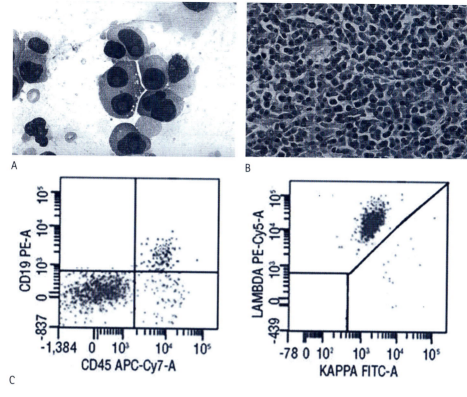

A

B

C

**Figure 33.1** Bone marrow plasma cell infiltrate in PCM. (A) The morphology of bone marrow aspirate (Geimsa, ×400); (B) histology of paraffin-embedded marrow trephine biopsy (hematoxylin and eosin, ×200); and (C) flow cytometry data demonstrating atypical plasma cells.

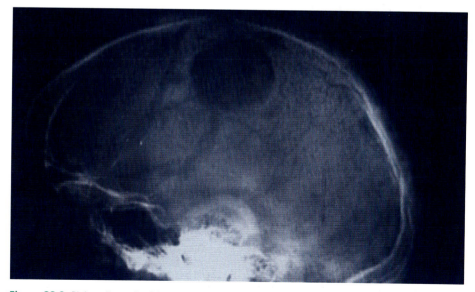

**Figure 33.2** Plain radiograph of the skull demonstrating characteristic lytic lesions.

### ASYMPTOMATIC MYELOMA (smouldering myeloma)

- M-protein level of ⩾30 g/l
- or bone marrow plasma cell infiltrate of ⩾10%
- No ROTI

### SYMPTOMATIC MYELOMA

- M-protein in serum or urine
- Bone marrow plasma cell infiltrate ⩽10%* or plasmacytoma
- Evidence of ROTI

*If flow cytometry confirms >90% neoplastic phenotype

### NON-SECRETORY MYELOMA

- No M-protein or detectable light chain excess
- Bone marrow plasma cell infiltrate ⩾10% or plasmacytoma
- Evidence of ROTI

**Figure 33.3** Definition of symptomatic/asymptomatic plasma cell myeloma.

# Recent Developments

The first clinically useful staging system utilizing a number of prognostic indicators reflecting tumour burden – the Durie–Salmon clinical staging system[3] – was devised in the early 1980s. This system, based on the presence of bone marrow failure, renal dysfunction and the extent of lytic bone disease, could separate patients prognostically into early stage disease (low tumour burden) with a median survival of 5 years and those with advanced stage disease (high tumour burden) with a median survival of 15 months. The addition of biological variables such as $\beta_2$-microglobulin ($\beta_2$-MG), C reactive protein (a surrogate indicator of interleukin-6 levels) and cytogenetic abnormalities may further refine this crude clinical staging system to allow the identification of those patients who will demonstrate the best response to conventional therapy. Abnormalities of chromo-

| Stage | Criteria | Median survival (months) |
|---|---|---|
| I | Serum $\beta_2$-MG <3.5 mg/l and serum albumin >35 g/l | 62 |
| II | Neither I nor III<br>Serum $\beta_2$-MG <3.5 mg/l and serum albumin <35 g/l<br>*or*<br>Serum $\beta_2$-MG 3.5–5.5 mg/l | 45 |
| III | Serum $\beta_2$-MG >5.5 mg/l | 29 |

**Figure 33.4** International Staging System.[4]

some 13 are associated with a poor prognosis. Recently a working group has devised, tested and validated an International Staging System (Figure 33.4) based on serum levels of $\beta_2$-MG and serum albumin, separating patients into three prognostic groups irrespective of the therapy used.[4] This system is simple and easily applied in clinical practice; however, the use of such a system to direct patient-specific therapy has not yet been adopted.

## Conclusion

The diagnosis of PCM has been refined over recent years, allowing clinicians to determine when to activate their treatment strategies. In addition, attempts to define prognostic groupings, and thus patients at greater risk of treatment failure, have resulted in the prognostic scoring systems based on clinical and surrogate biological markers of disease 'aggressiveness'. The impact of newer technological advances such as gene expression profiling or genetic polymorphism associations remains to be determined.

## Further Reading

1 Smith A, Wisloff F, Samson D. Guidelines on the diagnosis and management of multiple myeloma 2005. *Br J Haematol* 2006; **132**: 410–51.

2 Bradwell AR, Carr-Smith HD, Mead GP, Harvey TC, Drayson MT. Serum test for assessment of patients with Bence Jones myeloma. *Lancet* 2003; **361**: 489–91.

3 Durie BG, Salmon SE, Moon TE. Pretreatment tumor mass, cell kinetics, and prognosis in multiple myeloma. *Blood* 1980; **55**: 364–72.

4 Greipp PR, San Miguel J, Durie BG, *et al.* International staging system for multiple myeloma. *J Clin Oncol* 2005; **23**: 3412–20.

# 34 Myeloma – management

## Case History

A 46-year-old man presents with a pathological fracture of his left clavicle. He is diagnosed as suffering from plasma cell myeloma (PCM) based on a skeletal survey indicating multiple lytic lesions, serum electrophoresis revealing an immunoglobulin G (IgG) κ level of 54 g/l and a bone marrow infiltrate of 24% malignant plasma cells on diagnostic biopsy. He has one human leukocyte antigen (HLA)-identical sibling.

**What is the optimal management of the man's disease?**

**What is the role of allogeneic stem cell transplantation in his management strategy?**

**Where in his management should novel therapy be introduced?**

## Background

Prior to the introduction of alkylating agents, the median survival of patients with PCM was less than 1 year.[1] Approximately 60% of patients will respond to conventional chemotherapy, though approximately 25% of patients will be alive at 5 years and less than 10% will be alive at 10 years. The aim of therapy in patients with PCM is to control the disease process, to maximize quality of life and to prolong survival. Response criteria were first developed by the Committee of the Chronic Leukemia and Myeloma Task Force of the US National Cancer Institute in 1968, and were subsequently reviewed in 1973. In 1998, the Myeloma Subcommittee of the European Blood and Marrow Transplantation (EBMT) Chronic Leukaemia Working Party, in collaboration with the Myeloma Working Committee of the International Bone Marrow Transplant Registry, set out what have been universally adopted response criteria.[2] The main tenets are illustrated in Table 34.1. The published documents provide criteria for complete response (CR), partial response (PR), minimal response, stable disease, progressive disease, plateau response and relapse.

Most newly diagnosed patients below 65 years of age (or older if fit) are candidates for dose-escalation therapy including high-dose alkylating agent chemotherapy supported by autologous cryopreserved peripheral blood stem cells (autologous stem cell transplantation [ASCT]). Initial (induction) therapy must avoid agents with cumulative myelosuppressive side effects in order to permit collection of an adequate number of stem cells. Common pre-ASCT induction regimens have included high-dose dexamethasone alone or in combination with infusional vincristine, adriamycin (doxorubicin) and dexamethasone (VAD),[3] which can produce PR in 50%–60% of patients, with CR observed in

**Table 34.1** EBMT clinical response criteria.[2]

**Complete response (CR) requires all of the following:**

1. Absence of the original monoclonal paraprotein in serum and urine by immunofixation, maintained for a minimum of 6 weeks. The presence of oligoclonal bands consistent with oligoclonal immune reconstitution does not exclude CR.

2. <5% plasma cells in a bone marrow aspirate and also on trephine bone biopsy if biopsy is performed. If absence of monoclonal protein is sustained for 6 weeks it is not necessary to repeat the bone marrow examination, except in patients with non-secretory myeloma where the marrow examination must be repeated after an interval of at least 6 weeks to confirm CR.

3. No increase in size or number of lytic bone lesions (development of a compression fracture does not exclude response).

4. Disappearance of soft tissue plasmacytomas.

Patients in whom some, but not all, of the criteria for CR are fulfilled are classified as PR, providing the remaining criteria satisfy the requirements for PR. This includes patients in whom routine electrophoresis is negative but in whom immunofixation has not been performed.

**Partial response (PR) requires all of the following:**

1. ≥50% reduction in the level of the serum monoclonal paraprotein, maintained for a minimum of 6 weeks.

2. Reduction in 24-hour urinary light chain excretion either by ≥90% or to <200 mg, maintained for a minimum of 6 weeks.

3. For patients with non-secretory myeloma only, ≥50% reduction in plasma cells in a bone marrow aspirate and on trephine biopsy, if biopsy is performed, maintained for a minimum of 6 weeks.

4. ≥50% reduction in the size of soft tissue plasmacytomas (by radiography or clinical examination).

5. No increase in size or number of lytic bone lesions (development of a compression fracture does not exclude response).

Patients in whom some, but not all, of the criteria for PR are fulfilled are classified as MR, provided the remaining criteria satisfy the requirements for MR.

**Minimal response (MR) requires all of the following:**

1. 25%–49% reduction in the level of the serum monoclonal paraprotein maintained for a minimum of 6 weeks.

2. 50%–89% reduction in 24-hour urinary light chain excretion, which still exceeds 200 mg/24 hours, maintained for a minimum of 6 weeks.

3. For patients with non-secretory myeloma only, 25%–49% reduction in plasma cells in a bone marrow aspirate and on trephine biopsy if biopsy is performed, maintained for a minimum of 6 weeks.

4. 25%–49% reduction in the size of soft tissue plasmacytomas (by radiography or clinical examination).

5. No increase in the size or number of lytic bone lesions (development of a compression fracture does not exclude response). MR also includes patients in whom some, but not all, of the criteria for PR are fulfilled, provided the remaining criteria satisfy the requirements for MR.

**No change (NC)**

1. Not meeting the criteria of either minimal response or progressive disease.

**Plateau**

1. Stable values (within 25% above or below value at the time response is assessed) maintained for at least 3 months.

**Time point for assessing response**

1. Response to the transplant procedure will be assessed by comparison with results immediately prior to conditioning.

2. If transplant is part of a treatment programme, response to the whole treatment programme will be assessed by comparison with the results at the start of the programme.

**Relapse from CR requires at least one of the following:**

1. Reappearance of serum or urinary paraprotein on immunofixation or routine electrophoresis, confirmed by at least one further investigation and excluding oligoclonal immune reconstitution.

*continued*

**Table 34.1 Continued**

2. ≥5% plasma cells in a bone marrow aspirate or on trephine bone biopsy.

3. Development of new lytic bone lesions or soft tissue plasmacytomas or definite increase in the size of residual bone lesions (development of a compression fracture does not exclude continued response and may not indicate progression).

4. Development of hypercalcaemia (corrected serum calcium >11.5 mg/dl or 2.8 mmol/l) not attributable to any other cause.

**Progressive disease (for patients not in CR) requires one or more of the following:**

1. >25% increase in the level of the serum monoclonal paraprotein, which must also be an absolute increase of at least 5 g/l and confirmed by at least one repeated investigation.

2. >25% increase in the 24-hour urinary light chain excretion, which must also be an absolute increase of at least 200 mg/24 hours and confirmed by at least one repeated investigation.

3. >25% increase in plasma cells in a bone marrow aspirate or on trephine biopsy which must also be an absolute increase of at least 10%.

4. Definite increase in the size of existing bone lesions or soft tissue plasmacytomas.

5. Development of new bone lesions or soft tissue plasmacytomas (development of a compression fracture does not exclude continued response and may not indicate progression).

6. Development of hypercalcaemia (corrected serum calcium >11.5 mg/dl or 2.8 mmol/l) not attributable to any other cause.

5%–10% of patients. VAD and VAD hybrids achieve rapid, effective initial disease control and the addition of weekly cyclophosphamide has improved response rates without compromising the stem cell compartment.[4] The duration of induction therapy is usually 4–6 months, which achieves maximum response in the majority of patients who then can proceed with stem cell mobilization and ASCT.

Thalidomide, invented in the 1950s as a sedative anti-emetic, has demonstrated antimyeloma efficacy, particularly in the setting of advanced and refractory disease, and is only the third independently active compound for treating myeloma.[5] For induction therapy, the combination of thalidomide and dexamethasone has been demonstrated to be efficacious, producing higher rates of CR or near CR (nCR), and does not compromise stem cell collection or ASCT. Thalidomide regimens, particularly when given early in the disease course and in combination with chemotherapeutic agents, are associated with an increased toxicity, especially venous thromboembolism (VTE) events.[3] The precise mechanism of thalidomide-associated VTE is unknown, as is the best method for its prevention.

The use of stem cells (ASCT) to support the use of high-dose melphalan (140–200 mg/m$^2$) has become standard practice in the management of PCM.[4,6] A single ASCT after induction regimens typically produces CR in about 20%–40% of patients, with a median progression-free survival in the range of 2.5–4 years and overall survival of 4–5 years (Figure 34.1). Other studies in which transplantation was deferred until relapse have also suggested similar overall survival, although post-ASCT remissions were shorter compared with upfront ASCT. Factors that may predict the outcome of ASCT include a high $\beta_2$-microglobulin level at diagnosis and deletion of chromosome 13 (detected by conventional cytogenetics), which may confer a particularly poor prognosis.

In an attempt to improve the outcome of high-dose therapy, sequential administration of ASCT (tandem transplantation) has been advocated.[3] In a randomized control

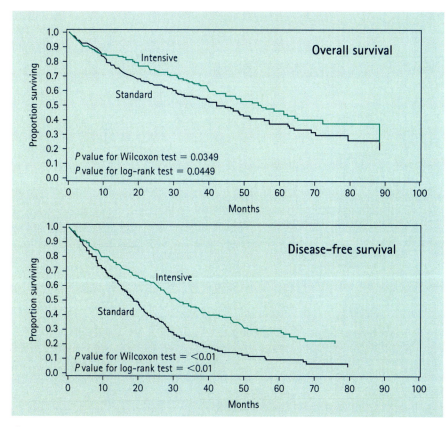

**Figure 34.1** Overall and disease-free survival advantage of high-dose therapy (Intensive) compared with conventional-dose chemotherapy (Standard) (with permission).[4]

study, the French Myeloma Group, IFM, reported an improved disease responsiveness and duration of response when a second ASCT was performed in those patients who failed to achieve a CR after the first ASCT.[7] Maintenance therapy after ASCT has remained an issue for many years and many agents have been used, including steroids, chemotherapy agents and interferon alfa. More recently, thalidomide has been used in the maintenance setting and whilst early results are encouraging, this approach is limited by toxicity.

Myeloablative allogeneic SCT (alloSCT) from a matched related donor can produce cure in a small proportion of selected patients but is limited by lack of appropriate donors, age limitations and significant risks of morbidity and mortality due to graft-versus-host disease and other complications. Although the 5-year survival rates may be comparable to ASCT, relapses after this time frame are much less frequent in the alloSCT-treated patients. More recently, reduced-intensity and non-myeloablative regimens have been explored in conditioning patients with PCM in order to mitigate some of the transplant-related mortality (TRM) while maintaining the graft-versus-myeloma (GvM) effect of alloSCT. Reduced-intensity conditioning (RIC) alloSCT has less early non-relapse mortality, although late relapses and transplant-related deaths have become

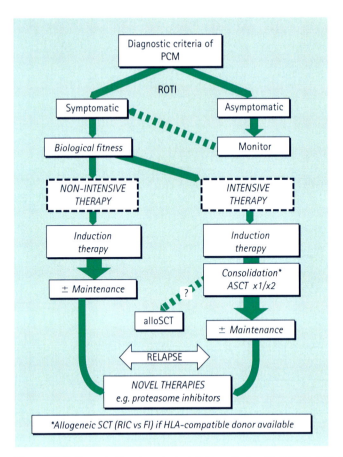

**Figure 34.2** Suggested treatment schedule for patients with PCM. FI, full intensity.

apparent.[3] As GvM is most likely to be successful in the setting of minimal residual disease, the prevailing opinion is for use of a tandem ASCT/RIC alloSCT and preliminary results indicate the feasibility and early efficacy of this approach. The use of alternative or unrelated donors in alloSCT for PCM is associated with significant TRM in the full-intensity setting but is improved using RIC regimens. Early experience with RIC matched unrelated donor alloSCT has suggested encouraging response and survival rates.[8] A suggested treatment algorithm is illustrated in Figure 34.2.

# Recent Developments

Through intense clinical research, a number of biological agents have been developed for use in PCM. Bortezomib (formerly PS341) specifically, selectively and reversibly inhibits the proteasome by binding tightly to the enzyme's active site. A number of trials using this drug in combination with other agents, such as dexamethasone, anthracyclines, alkylating agents (melphalan) and thalidomide, have been activated in newly diagnosed patients.[3] Overall response rates have been impressive, ranging from 75% to 100%, with

CR/nCR seen in 20%–30% of patients. The main side effects include diarrhoea, hypotension, fatigue, haematological toxicity and peripheral neuropathy (sensory and motor).

Immunomodulatory drugs (IMiDs) have now been shown to block several pathways important for disease progression in PCM. First established as agents with anti-angiogenic properties, IMiDs inhibit the production of interleukin-6, activate apoptotic pathways and activate T cells to produce interleukin-2. Lenalidomide is an IMiD that has also demonstrated efficacy, with a lower incidence of peripheral neuropathy, in relapsed/refractory myeloma patients.[9] Lenalidomide is approved by the US Food and Drug Administration and European Medicines Agency (EMEA) for use in combination with dexamethasone for the management of relapsed disease.

## Conclusion

Over the last 10 years, there has been a significant change in the management of young patients with PCM. The use of induction therapy followed by consolidation with high-dose therapy has been adopted as standard therapy. However, with the introduction of new, biological agents, the treatment strategies in PCM will be redesigned in the coming years.

## Further Reading

1 Korst DR, Clifford GO, Fowler WM, Louis J, Will J, Wilson HE. Multiple myeloma. II. Analysis of cyclophosphamide therapy in 165 patients. *JAMA* 1964; **189**: 758–62.

2 Bladé J, Samson D, Reece D, *et al.* Criteria for evaluating disease response and progression in patients with multiple myeloma treated by high-dose therapy and haemopoietic stem cell transplantation. Myeloma Subcommittee of the EBMT. European Group for Blood and Marrow Transplant. *Br J Haematol* 1998; **102**: 1115–23.

3 Barlogie B, Smith L, Alexanian R. Effective treatment of advanced multiple myeloma refractory to alkylating agents. *N Engl J Med* 1984; **310**: 1353–6.

4 Child JA, Morgan GJ, Davies FE, *et al.* High-dose chemotherapy with hematopoietic stem-cell rescue for multiple myeloma. *N Engl J Med* 2003; **348**: 1875–83.

5 Singhal S, Mehta J, Desikan R, *et al.* Antitumor activity of thalidomide in refractory multiple myeloma. *N Engl J Med* 1999; **341**: 1565–71.

6 Attal M, Harousseau JL, Stoppa AM, *et al.* A prospective, randomized trial of autologous bone marrow transplantation and chemotherapy in multiple myeloma. Intergroupe Français du Myélome. *N Engl J Med* 1996; **335**: 91–7.

7 Attal M, Harousseau JL, Facon T, *et al.* Single versus double autologous stem-cell transplantation for multiple myeloma. *N Engl J Med* 2003; **349**: 2495–502.

8 Smith A, Wisloff F, Samson D. Guidelines on the diagnosis and management of multiple myeloma 2005. *Br J Haematol* 2006; **132**: 410–51.

9 Richardson PG, Jagannath S, Schlossman R, *et al.* A multicenter, randomized, phase II study to evaluate the efficacy and safety of 2 CDC-5013 dose regimens when used alone or in combination with dexamethasone (Dex) for the treatment of relapsed or refractory multiple myeloma. *Blood* 2003; **102**: 235a.

# 35 Myeloma – treatment in the less fit or compromised patient

## Case History

A 74-year-old gentleman presented with tiredness and lethargy. He was found to be in renal failure with a serum creatinine level of 800 µmol/l and commenced on haemodialysis. He has a background of ischaemic heart disease, previous coronary artery bypass grafting and emphysema. Further investigations revealed an immunoglobulin G (IgG) κ paraprotein of 32 g/l with reduction in IgA and IgM levels.

**What treatment is most appropriate for this patient?**

**Is there a role for plasma exchange in patients with renal failure secondary to plasma cell myeloma (PCM)?**

**What are the different aspects of supportive care?**

## Background

Not all patients with PCM are potential candidates for dose-escalation programmes, including autologous stem cell transplantation. The aim of therapy in these patients is to achieve disease control with minimal side effects, inducing improved quality of life. Melphalan and prednisone (MP) has been the mainstay of treatment in such patients and yields partial remission in 50%–55% of cases, with only occasional complete remission.[1] Prednisone has been replaced with dexamethasone and directly compared to MP. The response rates were similar but there was considerably greater toxicity associated with dexamethasone.[2,3] Cyclophosphamide is efficacious, especially when used in combination with steroids. Other combinations of alkylating agents, such as VBMCP (vincristine, carmustine, melphalan, cyclophosphamide and prednisone), have been utilized and, more recently, thalidomide has been added to MP with improved response rates but increased toxicity.[4] The aim of MP therapy is to deliver maximum response followed by 3 months of therapy and, to date, no randomized study has shown a benefit to prolonging therapy beyond this time frame. The introduction of thalidomide to MP may alter this time frame, especially the notion of following maximum response to MP plus thalidomide with thalidomide monotherapy as a maintenance strategy, and is currently under investigation.

### The approach to acute renal failure and the role of plasmapheresis

Plasma cell myeloma is associated with renal dysfunction in up to 50% of patients, with renal failure occurring in a significant proportion of patients. The presence of renal dysfunction/failure is associated with higher treatment- and disease-related mortality and limits clinical decision making when designing patient treatment strategies. The characteristic histopathological feature on renal biopsy is the 'myeloma kidney' or cast nephropathy due to excessive amounts of filtered intraluminal toxic light chains. Other causes of renal failure include hypercalcaemia, infection, dehydration and nephrotoxic drugs. General approaches to treat renal failure in myeloma include vigorous hydration, avoidance of toxins and nephrotoxic drugs, and aggressive treatment of infections and hypercalcaemia. However, these measures are often inadequate to reverse oliguric and advanced renal failure. Several case reports showed benefit from plasma exchange by acutely reducing levels of the light chain protein.[5] So far, randomized studies have failed to demonstrate a significant benefit from plasmapheresis in this setting,[6] though the clinical impact of such a strategy may be masked by the limited sample sizes. Ongoing studies such as the UKMF MERIT trial are attempting to answer the plasma exchange question.

# Recent Developments

## 1. Supportive care – erythropoietin

Many patients present with anaemia (haemoglobin [Hb] <10 g/dl) either as a result of disease infiltration of the marrow, tumour-associated cytokine production or renal dysfunction or related to chemotherapy or a combination of these scenarios. Erythropoietin (EPO) therapy has been utilized in patients with multiple myeloma and can induce a response, as defined by a rise in the Hb of >2 g/dl, in approximately 70% of patients, though results are best in those who have not been exposed to alkylating chemotherapeutic agents.[7] The current guidelines of the UK Myeloma Forum and Nordic Myeloma Study Group suggest that EPO should not be used in newly diagnosed patients until the initial response to chemotherapy has been determined, though a therapeutic trial in symptomatic patients can be tried.[8] High serum EPO (>200 IU/ml), a high transfusion requirement for packed red cells and a low platelet count are negative prognostic indicators of response to EPO.

## 2. Assessment of infective risk

The risk of infection in patients with PCM at diagnosis or during treatment is not insignificant, resulting from a combination of both cellular and humoral immune defects and the direct immuno- and myelosuppression of the treatment strategies. The risk of infection is highest in the first 3 months after diagnosis but decreases with response to antimyeloma therapy. Prompt access of febrile patients to specialist medical assessment is recommended to promote rapid administration of appropriate antimicrobial therapy. Patients presenting with a febrile illness need to be treated with broad-spectrum intravenous antibiotics. The prevention of infection in patients with PCM undergoing treatment has improved the overall outlook. The use of prophylactic immunoglobulin infusions (0.4 g/kg body weight) may be helpful, especially for those in plateau-phase disease. Prophylactic antibiotics are not recommended except for the regular use of trimethoprim–sulphamethoxazole in the first 2–3 months from diagnosis. Vaccinations against influenza, *Streptococcus pneumoniae* and *Haemophilus influenzae* are recommended but the efficacy is likely to be limited given the established immune-cell dysfunction associated with myeloma.[8]

### 3. Bisphosphonates

Bisphosphonates are stable analogues of inorganic pyrophosphates that are taken up by osteoclasts and inhibit their activity, maturation and survival. Due to their ability to inhibit bone resorption, bisphosphonates play an important role in the supportive care of patients with PCM not only in the treatment of hypercalcaemia but also by reducing the incidence of skeletal complications. New-generation bisphosphonates such as pamidronate and zoledronic acid are up to 100 fold more potent than first-generation compounds such as etidronate or clodronate. Studies have shown that intravenous pamidronate (90 mg) given every three to four weeks significantly reduces the incidence and delays the onset of skeletal-related events compared with placebo.[9] Serious adverse events are infrequent but doses have to be adjusted in patients with renal impairment. Osteonecrosis of the jaw has been reported in particular with zoledronic acid.

## Conclusion

With the heterogeneity of the disease progression and the spectrum of biological performance of patients with PCM, tailor-made treatment strategies are essential. In particular, supportive care to limit disease- and therapy-related complications is essential if improved quality of life is the goal of treatment.

## Further Reading

1 Myeloma Trialists' Collaborative Group. Combination chemotherapy versus melphalan plus prednisone as treatment for multiple myeloma: an overview of 6,633 patients from 27 randomized trials. *J Clin Oncol* 1998; **16**: 3832–42.

2 Greipp PR, San Miguel J, Durie BG, *et al.* International staging system for multiple myeloma. *J Clin Oncol* 2005; **23**: 3412–20.

3 Hernández JM, Garcïa-Sanz R, Golvano E, *et al.* Randomized comparison of dexamethasone combined with melphalan versus melphalan with prednisone in the treatment of elderly patients with multiple myeloma. *Br J Haematol* 2004; **127**: 159–64.

4 Palumbo A, Bertola A, Musto P, *et al.* A prospective randomized trial of oral melphalan, prednisone, thalidomide (MPT) vs oral melphalan, prednisone (MP): an interim analysis. *Blood* 2004; **104**: 207.

5 El-Achkar TM, Sharfuddin AA, Dominguez J. Approach to acute renal failure with multiple myeloma: role of plasmapheresis. *Ther Apher Dial* 2005; **9**: 417–22.

6 Clark WF, Stewart AK, Rock GA, *et al.* Plasma exchange when myeloma presents as acute renal failure: a randomized, controlled trial. *Ann Intern Med* 2005; **143**: 777–84.

7 Cazzola M, Beguin Y, Kloczko J, Spicka I, Coiffier B. Once-weekly epoetin beta is highly effective in treating anaemic patients with lymphoproliferative malignancy and defective endogenous erythropoietin production. *Br J Haematol* 2003; **122**: 386–93.

8 Smith A, Wisloff F, Samson D. Guidelines on the diagnosis and management of multiple myeloma 2005. *Br J Haematol* 2006; **132**: 410–51.

9 Saad F. Zoledronic acid: past, present and future roles in cancer treatment. *Future Oncol* 2005; **1**: 149–59.

# 36 Myeloma – solitary plasmacytoma

## Case History

A 74-year-old female noticed a swelling on her anterior chest wall for several months, gradually increasing in size. More recently it became painful and prompted her to see her General Practitioner. She has no other symptoms.

**Which investigations should be performed to exclude myeloma?**

**What treatment options are most appropriate?**

**How likely is it that she will progress to myeloma?**

## Background

Solitary plasmacytomas are relatively rare and represent only 5% of patients with plasma cell dyscrasias. They present either in the bone or as an extramedullary mass. Some will present with a painful/symptomatic lesion (Figure 36.1) whilst others will be picked up during radiological examination for either an unrelated disease or during the investigation of a monoclonal immunoglobulin.[1] Solitary bone plasmacytomas (SBP) have a high risk of progression to multiple myeloma and, with the introduction of magnetic resonance imaging (MRI), it is apparent that up to 25% of patients originally labelled as having SBP will in fact have disease elsewhere.[2] Extramedullary plasmacytomas (EP) are, in contrast, almost always localized and have a high cure rate with radiotherapy. The median age of presentation with plasmacytoma is in the mid-fifth decade, a little younger than multiple myeloma, and there is a male predominance.[3]

Histological diagnosis should include identification of monoclonal plasma cells with appropriate immunohistochemical staining, such as staining for CD138 and κ/λ proteins to demonstrate monoclonal plasma cells. Other useful markers usually employed are MUM1/IRF4, CD56, CD117, CD27 and cyclin D1. To confidently diagnose a SBP there must be a single lytic lesion on skeletal survey and no evidence of systemic myeloma or related end-organ tissue damage (myeloma-related organ and/or tissue impairment; ROTI). Traditionally there should also be no evidence of plasma cell infiltrate in the bone marrow; however, more sensitive techniques are now demonstrating very low-level infiltrates present in a proportion of cases. All patients should be fully assessed to exclude multiple myeloma.[4] Solitary bone plasmacytomas primarily affect the axial skeleton and vertebrae.

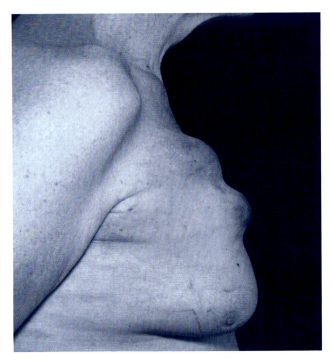

**Figure 36.1** Extramedullary plasmacytoma in the subdermal plane of the anterior thorax.

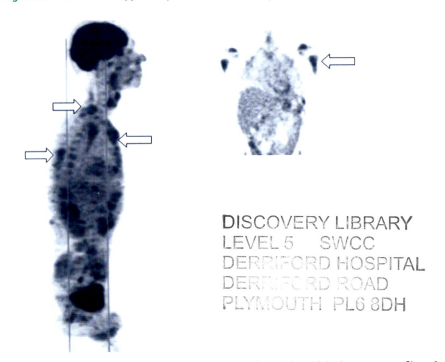

**Figure 36.2** Positron emission tomography image of a patient with multiple plasmacytomas. Sites of disease activity are indicated by arrows.

# Recent Developments

The role of sensitive imaging techniques is becoming apparent and MRI, computed tomography or positron emission tomography imaging (Figure 36.2) to detect occult lesions not shown on plain radiography is certainly desirable and should be performed wherever possible.[5]

The monoclonal serum component is variable in patients with SBP but can be detected in up to 72% of cases. In EP, the quoted incidence is much lower at less than 25%. The levels of serum monoclonal immunoglobulins do, however, tend to be lower than those seen in multiple myeloma and Bence–Jones proteinuria is less common.[4]

Extramedullary plasmacytomas occur more commonly in the respiratory sinuses and upper respiratory tract (>80%) alongside the gastrointestinal tract[1] but are also seen in the skin, lymph nodes, thymus and at almost any other site.[6,7] It is important to exclude bone destruction, occult disease at distant sites and soft tissue spread of multiple myeloma before making the diagnosis.

## Treatment

### Solitary plasmacytoma of bone

Local radiotherapy is the mainstay of treatment, although there is no consensus in the literature for the most appropriate dosing schedule. There is at present little evidence to back the use of bisphosphonates in the management of SBP. Patients with more extensive disease should be treated as for multiple myeloma.

### Solitary extramedullary plasmacytomas

Radiotherapy should follow the same guidance as that for solitary plasmacytomas of bone. However, if cervical nodes are involved, as is the case in 10%–40% of upper respiratory or upper gastrointestinal disease,[8] then these should be included in the radiotherapy field. Surgery is not generally recommended for the treatment of head and neck EP but should be considered at other sites if complete removal of the tumour is feasible. In the rare cases of relapsed/refractory/progressive disease, cytotoxic treatment should be considered.[4]

# Conclusion

Solitary plasmacytoma of bone will, in the majority of patients, progress to multiple myeloma after a median of 2–4 years, with a median overall survival of 7–12 years. Between 15% and 45% of patients treated will, however, remain disease free at 10 years; this group is likely to be those in whom paraprotein concentrations become unrecordable within the first year post-treatment (implying the disease was fully eradicated with radiotherapy) rather than those with either persisting monoclonal immunoglobulins or non-secretory disease.[7] Extramedullary plasmacytomas are very radiosensitive and local control is usually achieved in over 80% of patients, with between 50% and 65% of those remaining disease free at 10 years. For those patients who do progress to multiple myeloma, this occurs after a median of 1.5–2.5 years and the prognosis at this point appears to be similar to those with *de novo* disease.

# Further Reading

1 Kyle RA. Monoclonal gammopathy of undetermined significance and solitary plasmacytoma. Implications for progression to overt multiple myeloma. *Hematol Oncol Clin North Am* 1997; **11**: 71–87.

2 Moulopoulos LA, Dimopoulos MA, Weber D, Fuller L, Libshitz HI, Alexanian R. Magnetic resonance imaging in the staging of solitary plasmacytoma of bone. *J Clin Oncol* 1993; **11**: 1311–15.

3 Dimopoulos MA, Moulopoulos LA, Maniatis A, Alexanian R. Solitary plasmacytoma of bone and asymptomatic multiple myeloma. *Blood* 2000; **96**: 2037–44.

4 Soutar R, Lucraft H, Jackson G, *et al.* Guidelines on the diagnosis and management of solitary plasmacytoma of bone and solitary extramedullary plasmacytoma. *Br J Haematol* 2004; **124**: 717–26.

5 Smith A, Wisloff F, Samson D. Guidelines on the diagnosis and management of multiple myeloma 2005. *Br J Haematol* 2006; **132**: 410–51.

6 Dimopoulos MA, Hamilos G. Solitary bone plasmacytoma and extramedullary plasmacytoma. *Curr Treat Options Oncol* 2002; **3**: 255–9.

7 Wilder RB, Ha CS, Cox JD, Weber D, Delasalle K, Alexanian R. Persistence of myeloma protein for more than one year after radiotherapy is an adverse prognostic factor in solitary plasmacytoma of bone. *Cancer* 2002; **94**: 1532–7.

8 Hu K, Yahalom J. Radiotherapy in the management of plasma cell tumors. *Oncology (Williston Park)* 2000; **14**: 101–108,111; discussion 111–12, 115.

# 37 Myeloma – AL amyloid

## Case History

A 57-year-old woman presents with nephrotic syndrome and renal dysfunction. Investigation reveals a serum free light chain excess and a modest bone marrow infiltration with malignant phenotype plasma cells. Imaging reveals her to have enlarged kidneys and a rectal biopsy reveals amyloid deposits stained with Congo red.

**What further assessments and investigations are appropriate?**

**What is the optimal management of the woman's disease?**

**What is the role of stem cell transplantation in the management of amyloid?**

## Background

*Amyloidosis* describes a group of conditions characterized by the deposition of extracellular protein molecules in an ordered structure to make linear fibrils 7.5–10 nm wide arranged in characteristic β-sheets. These β-sheets produce apple-green birefringence under polarized light when stained with Congo red. Amyloidosis was first reported in 1854 by Virchow and he coined the name due to the apparent affinity of the protein material for iodine.[1] Originally, the amyloidoses were classified as either primary (occurring in those with no underlying pathology) or secondary (occurring in those with chronic inflammation or infection). However, with the discovery that several different proteins could cause amyloidosis, the revised categorization is based on the protein precursor, as illustrated in Table 37.1. AL amyloidosis is the commonest form, which is a protein conformation disorder associated with a clonal plasma cell dyscrasia.[2] Multiple organ disease results from the deposition of monoclonal immunoglobulin light chain fragments in insoluble fibrils, which associate *in vivo* with the normal plasma protein serum amyloid P (SAP) component, and the accumulation of the fibrils progressively disrupts the normal tissue structure leading to organ dysfunction, e.g. of the kidneys, heart and liver. Deposition of the amyloid fibrils evokes little or no local reaction in the tissues.

AL amyloidosis is a progressive and fatal disease, often (in about 80% of patients) within 2 years.[3] Therapy is aimed at reducing the light chain production, resulting in the stabilization or regression of existing amyloid deposits, and can be associated with improvement in end-organ function. AL amyloidosis may be associated with plasma cell myeloma (PCM) or other B-cell malignancies, and coexistent AL amyloid deposits are identified either at presentation or at some time during the course of PCM in approxi-

**Table 37.1 Nomenclature and classification of amyloid and amyloidoses**

| Amyloid type | Protein precursor | Protein type or variant | Associated clinical syndromes |
|---|---|---|---|
| AL | κ, λ | Aκ, Aλ | Primary amyloidosis, plasma cell myeloma, Waldenström's macroglobulinaemia |
| AH | IgG1 | Aγ1 | Heavy chain disease associated |
| AA | ApoSAA | AA | Reactive/secondary amyloidosis |
| | | | Familial Mediterranean fever |
| ATTR | Transthyretin | Met30 | Hereditary amyloidosis: |
| | | Met111 | Familial amyloidotic polyneuropathies |
| | | | Familial amyloidotic cardiomyopathy |
| AApoAl | Apolipoprotein A-I | Arg26 | Familial amyloidotic polyneuropathy |
| | | Arg60 | Ostertag-type familial amyloidosis |
| Agel | Gelsolin | Asn187 | Finnish-type familial amyloidosis |
| Aβ$_2$-m | β$_2$-microglobulin | | Dialysis associated |
| Aβ | β-protein precursor A4 | β A4 protein | Alzheimer's disease, Down's syndrome |
| | | Gln695 | Hereditary cerebral haemorrhage with amyloid (Dutch) |
| Acys | Cystatin-C | Leu68 | Hereditary cerebral haemorrhage with amyloid (Icelandic) |
| Ascr | PrP$^c$ | PrP$^c$, PrP$^{CJD}$ | Spongiform encephalopathies |
| Acal | (Pro)calcitonin | (Pro)calcitonin | Medullary carcinoma of thyroid |
| AANF | Atrial natriuretic factor | Atrial natriuretic factor | Isolated atrial amyloidosis |
| AIAPP | Islet-associated peptide | Islet-associated peptide | Amyloid of the islets, diabetes mellitus type II |
| A Lys | Lysozyme | Thr56 | Hereditary non-neuropathic systemic amyloidosis |
| A Fib | Fibrinogen α chain | Leu554 | Hereditary renal amyloidosis |

Data from: WHO-IUIS Nomenclature Sub-Committee. Nomenclature of amyloid and amyloidoses. *Bull World Health Organ* 1993; 71: 105–12.

mately 10%–15% of patients and more rarely in Waldenström's macroglobulinaemia. It is rare for AL amyloidosis to progress to overt PCM, presumably because of the short survival of patients with AL amyloidosis.

The age-adjusted incidence of AL amyloidosis in the USA is estimated to be between 5.1 and 12.8 per million persons per year,[4] which is equivalent to approximately 600 new cases per year in the UK. AL amyloidosis is estimated to be the cause of death in 1/1500 deaths in the UK. Approximately 60%–70% of patients are aged between 50 and 70 years of age at diagnosis, with less than 10% being below 50 years of age, and the male:female ratio is equal.

**Table 37.2** Clinical manifestations of end-organ involvement with amyloidosis

| Organ system | Frequency | Histopathology | Clinical features and symptoms |
|---|---|---|---|
| Kidney | ~33% | Glomerular lesion causing marked proteinuria and nephrotic syndrome | • Mild renal dysfunction is frequent, progressive renal failure is uncommon<br>• Ankle swelling, fatigue and loss of energy<br>• Body cavity effusions (pericardial, pleural, peritoneal)<br>• Orthostatic hypotension |
| Cardiac | ~20% | Amyloid deposition resulting in restrictive cardiomyopathy | • Abnormalities on a 12-lead electrocardiogram – low voltage changes<br>• Clinical signs of right-sided heart failure or those associated with a low cardiac output<br>• Orthostatic hypotension<br>• Atrial thrombi and atrial fibrillation<br>• Restrictive cardiomyopathy |
| Nervous system | ~20% | Amyloid deposition resulting in nerve conduction defects | • Polyneuropathy may give rise to parasthesiae and muscle weakness<br>• Sensory neuropathy is usually symmetrical, affecting the lower extremities, and may be painful<br>• Motor neuropathy is rare<br>• Carpal tunnel syndrome is common<br>• Autonomic neuropathy giving rise to postural hypotension, impotence and disturbed gastrointestinal (GI) motility<br>• Postural hypotension (fall in systolic blood pressure of at least 20 mmHg when a patient has been standing for 3–5 min after spending at least 5 min supine) |
| GI tract | 10%–25% | Mucosal/submucosal amyloid deposition | • Focal or diffuse with symptoms relating to the site of involvement<br>• Macroglossia and occasionally obstructive airways symptoms and sleep apnoea<br>• Diarrhoea, chronic nausea, malabsorption and weight loss<br>• GI perforation or haemorrhage<br>• Hepatomegaly |
| Haemostatic | ~33%–50% | Endothelial amyloid deposition distorting vessel contractibility | • Haemostatic screen abnormalities<br>• Commonest manifestation of bleeding is purpura, e.g. peri-orbital purpura ('raccoon eyes')<br>• Life-threatening bleeding potential, particularly GI |
| Localized | | Focal infiltrate of clonal lymphoplasmacytoid cells | • Upper respiratory (vocal cords) and pulmonary infiltration<br>• Musculoskeletal (arthropathy)<br>• Urogenital<br>• Adrenal and thyroid glands<br>• GI tract<br>• Skin<br>• Localized disease is not usually associated with measurable paraprotein or serum free light chains |

The most common clinical features at diagnosis are:

1  nephrotic syndrome with or without renal insufficiency;
2  congestive cardiomyopathy;
3  sensorimotor and/or autonomic peripheral neuropathy;
4  hepatomegaly.

Whilst systemic symptoms of fatigue and weight loss may be common, they are rarely presenting features and patients generally present with one particular organ that is dysfunctional. Clinical characteristics are illustrated in Table 37.2.

Confirmation of the diagnosis of amyloidosis is provided through tissue histology and should include serial investigations to determine the extent of disease. Amyloid deposits stain with Congo red and produce pathognomonic apple-green birefringence under cross-polarized light microscopy. A full investigation to determine the presence of a monoclonal plasma cell dyscrasia should be undertaken, as described in earlier chapters. A paraprotein is detectable in the serum or urine by routine electrophoresis in approximately 50% of patients, although the level is <10 g/l in 30% of patients. As such, immunofixation is recommended to increase sensitivity of detection. Serum free light chains can now be detected and quantitated in 98% of patients.[5,6] Radiolabelled SAP component localizes to amyloid deposits in proportion to the quantity of amyloid present, enabling the quantification of deposits by whole-body scintigraphy, although cardiac amyloid is poorly visualized.[7]

AL amyloidosis is associated with a poor prognosis; fewer than 5% of all AL amyloidosis patients survive ten or more years from the time of diagnosis.[3] A poor prognosis is associated with cardiac involvement, widespread deposition as determined by SAP scintigraphy, autonomic neuropathy and hepatic involvement. As yet, there is no specific therapy to augment the removal of amyloid fibrils and therefore treatment strategies are aimed at reducing or even stopping amyloid production whilst providing supportive care for organ dysfunction. Chemotherapy regimens used in AL amyloidosis are based on those that have proved to be effective in patients with PCM. Whilst slow-acting regimens may not impact the disease process, given the limited overall survival, high-dose therapy regimens are associated with a high procedural risk compared to patients with PCM, as a result of multiorgan involvement.

Single-agent melphalan or cyclophosphamide (with or without prednisolone) is appropriate, and symptomatic benefit can be seen in about 20%–30% of patients after a median of 12 months. Monthly courses of VAD (vincristine, adriamycin [doxorubicin] and dexamethasone)/VAD-hybrids or intravenous intermediate-dose melphalan (25 mg/m$^2$) with or without dexamethasone have been used. Caution over augmenting amyloid-associated cardiac dysfunction through the use of anthracyclines should be noted and the use of high-dose steroids can be complicated by severe fluid retention. Thalidomide may be useful in combination as initial therapy but caution over exacerbation of known thalidomide side effects in amyloidosis should be noted given the systemic nature of the disease. Colchicine may be effective in the treatment of AA amyloidosis complicating familial Mediterranean fever but has no role in AL amyloidosis. Experience of autologous stem cell transplantation (ASCT; melphalan 100–200 mg/m$^2$) in AL amyloidosis extends 10 years and can result in reversal of the clinical manifestations in up to approximately 60% of patients who survive the procedure.[8] This is associated with regression of AL amyloid deposits, reduction/elimination of clonal plasma cells and improved quality of life. However, the transplant-related mortality (TRM) is higher than for patients with PCM, ranging up to 40%.[7] The causes of death included cardiac arrhythmias, intractable hypotension, multiorgan failure and gastrointestinal (GI) bleeding. Patients with poor renal function and those who are already dialysis dependent perform particularly badly.[8] There is also a significant risk, including death, associated with stem cell mobilization in patients with AL amyloidosis.[8] The role of ASCT therefore remains unclear and it is reasonable to restrict ASCT to younger patients with one or two involved organs, who have not had previous amyloid-related GI bleeding, who do not have severe cardiomyopathy or advanced renal failure or who are not dialysis dependent. A small proportion of patients may derive significant clinical benefit from allogeneic stem cell transplantation (alloSCT), though given the TRM of full-intensity protocols, reduced-intensity conditioning alloSCT is currently under investigation.

Patients with end-stage renal failure should be considered for dialysis and renal transplantation may be a suitable option for selected patients. In patients with cardiac involvement, congestive cardiac failure should be treated predominantly with diuretics; angiotensin converting enzyme inhibitors should be used with caution and calcium-channel blockers and β-blockers are best avoided. Digoxin is generally contraindicated in patients with cardiac involvement and in patients where cardiac manifestations are the predominant or only signs/symptoms of amyloidosis; cardiac transplantation may be considered but this procedure should be followed by chemotherapy treatment to prevent reaccumulation of amyloid in the transplanted heart. In patients who experience orthostatic hypotension, the use of support stockings coupled with modest doses of fludrocortisone can be effective in selected patients. Midodrine is the most effective drug for orthostatic hypotension in patients with amyloidosis, but can cause supine hypertension and should be used with caution.

# Recent Developments

Anti-amyloid antibodies are currently undergoing phase I and II clinical trials as they might enhance clearance of amyloid deposits. R-1-[6-[R-2-carboxy-pyrrolidin-1-yl]-6-oxo-hexanoyl]pyrrolidine-2-carboxylic acid (CPHPC) is a drug currently developed to inhibit the binding of SAP to amyloid fibrils. Mouse experiments showed rapid reduction of plasma SAP concentration. This drug is now under investigation in open-label studies to examine the tolerability, safety and efficacy of CPHPC in patients with systemic amyloidosis.[9]

# Conclusion

Recent advances in understanding the mechanisms of amyloid production have identified several novel therapeutic targets. Hopefully, these new therapeutic strategies will be effective in a wide spectrum of disorders ranging from systemic amyloidosis to Alzheimer's disease and maturity-onset diabetes.

# Further Reading

1 Friedreich N, Kekulé A. Zur Amyloidfrage. *Virchows Archiv A. Pathological Anatomy* 1859; **16**.

2 Falk RH, Comenzo RL, Skinner M. The systemic amyloidoses. *N Engl J Med* 1997; **337**: 898–909.

3 Kyle RA, Gertz MA, Greipp PR, *et al.* Long-term survival (10 years or more) in 30 patients with primary amyloidosis. *Blood* 1999; **93**: 1062–6.

4 Kyle RA, Linos A, Beard CM, *et al*. Incidence and natural history of primary systemic amyloidosis in Olmsted County, Minnesota, 1950 through 1989. *Blood* 1992; **79**: 1817–22.

5 Bradwell AR, Carr-Smith HD, Mead GP, *et al*. Highly sensitive, automated immunoassay for immunoglobulin free light chains in serum and urine. *Clin Chem* 2001; **47**: 673–80.

6 Lachmann HJ, Gallimore R, Gillmore JD, *et al*. Outcome in systemic AL amyloidosis in relation to changes in concentration of circulating free immunoglobulin light chains following chemotherapy. *Br J Haematol* 2003; **122**: 78–84.

7 Bird J, Cavenagh J, Hawkins P, Lachmann H, Mehta A, Samson D. Guidelines on the diagnosis and management of AL amyloidosis. *Br J Haematol* 2004; **125**: 681–700.

8 Comenzo RL, Gertz MA. Autologous stem cell transplantation for primary systemic amyloidosis. *Blood* 2002; **99**: 4276–82.

9 Gillmore JD, Hawkins PN. Drug insight: emerging therapies for amyloidosis. *Nature Clinical Practice Nephrology* 2006: **2**: 263–270.

# Index